See It! I

FITNEVISION

Get A Fit Mind and A Fit Body

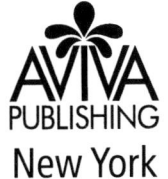

AVIVA
PUBLISHING
New York

Sandi Berger C.F.T., L.C.
Certified Fitness Trainer and Life Coach

FITNEVISION: Get A Fit Mind and A Fit Body

Copyright © 2012 Sandi Berger

All rights reserved. No part of this book may be reproduced, stored in a retrieval system, or transmitted by any means, electronic, mechanical, photocopying, recording, or otherwise, without written permission from the publisher.

Address all inquiries to:
Sandi Berger
www.Fitnevision.com

Library of Congress Control Number: Applied for.

ISBN: 978-1-935586-68-5

Editor: Tyler Tichelaar

Cover Design & Interior Layout: Fusion Creative Works,
www.fusioncw.com

Aviva Publishing, New York

For additional copies visit: www.Fitnevision.com

DEDICATION

I dedicate *FITNEVISION* to my parents,
Burt and Louise Berger.

I thank my dad for his entrepreneurial spirit, his talent for percussion (drums) and dance, and for his style. And for his silly sense of humor—for that gene is the most important one for being able to look at life and laugh!

I thank my mom for giving me the gene of internal strength and a positive outlook on life. You were a woman ahead of your time, but unfortunately, I did not recognize your gifts until after your death.

Love to you both wherever your spirits may be!

~ Your daughter, Sandi

CONTENTS

Introduction: Welcome to *FITNEVISION*	7
PART I: SEE IT! BELIEVE IT! SEIZE IT! BECOME IT!	**13**
Chapter 1: *FITNEVISION*: Body and Mind Fitness	15
Chapter 2: Keeping a Journal	29
Chapter 3: How Your Visions Affect Others	35
Chapter 4: Living Life with Passion	45
Chapter 5: Creating Your Emotional Toolbox	53
Chapter 6: Being Unique	59
Chapter 7: The Yin and the Yang Inside	65
Chapter 8: Dancing	71
Chapter 9: What Is Your Purpose for Being on this Planet?	77
Chapter 10: Birds of a Feather Usually Share a Similar Vision	83
Chapter 11: Goal Setting Is Part of Creating Your *FITNEVISION*	89
Chapter 12: Fake It and Watch Yourself Make It	95
Chapter 13: One Choice Away from a Fabulous Life	101
Chapter 14: Trust in Faith and Mazel	109
Chapter 15: If You Don't Like You, No One Else Will	115
Chapter 16: F.E.A.R. and Other Lies We Tell Ourselves	123
Chapter 17: C.A.N.E.L. (Constant And Never-Ending Learning)	131
Chapter 18: Getting in Touch with Your Cast of Characters	139
Chapter 19: Change What You See and You Change What You Get	149
Chapter 20: You are the Ultimate Driving Machine—Inside and Out	155
Chapter 21: Eat Healthy: What You Put in Your Body Determines Your Performance	161
Chapter 22: Getting in Touch with Your Disowned Self	167
Chapter 23: Falling in Love with You	177

Chapter 24: In Real Estate, It's All about Location, Location, Location. In Managing a Healthy Lifestyle, It's All about Discipline, Discipline, Discipline.	183
Chapter 25: It's Not Just Fitness. It's a Lifestyle Package.	189
Chapter 26: You Reap What You S.E.W.	195
Chapter 27: Accepting Yourself Right Here, Right Now!	203
Chapter 28: Connecting with Yourself and Others	211
Chapter 29: The Wills, Won'ts, and Can'ts	219
Chapter 30: SEE IT! BELIEVE IT! SEIZE IT! BECOME IT!	225
Chapter 31: Freedom to Be You Starts with Honesty	231
Chapter 32: "Blissipline"—The Power of a Positive Attitude	237
Chapter 33: Failure Is Not Being Overweight. Failure Is Staying Overweight.	243
Chapter 34: Fire Your Therapist and Get on the Vision Plan	249
Chapter 35: Ready, Set, Visualize!	257
Chapter 36: Putting It All Together	261
PART II: *FITNEVISION* AND MY PERSONAL JOURNEY	**263**
Chapter 1: My Personal Experience: Attack of the Aliens	265
Chapter 2: Closets are for Clothes	273
Chapter 3: The Great Depression of 1975	279
Chapter 4: Fifty Cents a Pack	285
Chapter 5: Learning How to Drive a Stick Shift	291
Chapter 6: Hip, Hip, Hooray! For Author Louise Hay	297
Chapter 7: Learning from Others	303
Chapter 8: Amazing Grace	309
A Final Note	315
A Call to Action	317
About the Author	319
Book Sandi Berger	321

INTRODUCTION: WELCOME TO *FITNEVISION*

The mere fact that you have selected to read this book tells me that you have tried a lot of different strategies and techniques to become your best self, but you are still searching for that right ingredient. Guess what? You will never just learn one way to be your best self. But *FITNEVISION* is an additional tool you can use to assist and guide you on your journey toward health and happiness.

This book is divided into two sections: Part One contains some techniques and strategies for creating your *FITNEVISION* Lifestyle Program. Part Two is based on some of my personal experiences. I offer these experiences as examples of how, with the power of vision, I overcame obstacles in my path to becoming a healthier human being. When I read a book with an author's real life experiences, I learn faster, and I can get results a lot quicker because the author's experiences teach me what "not" to do. We are all students and teachers of how to live. We teach each other all the time. We all learn from others' experiences so I want to share mine to help my readers.

But I'll do more than share. I'll give you ideas to act upon—activities to do to help make your *FITNEVISION* come true. At times, I may sound repetitive or ask you to do things I already asked you to do earlier in the book. That is intentional on my part because our brains learn through repetition. We need to process and reprogram our minds toward making healthy and happy choices for ourselves, and we do that by memorizing positive affirmations and repeating positive activities. So even if it feels like you're doing the same thing over and over, do it with a happy mindset and remember that practice makes perfect.

It's important, also, that you read and work through this book slowly. Don't rush. The purpose of *FITNEVISION* is not to prove to yourself that you are a speed reader. The purpose is not for you to check off one more book you have read. You will have a reading experience here, yes, but more importantly, you want to have a life-changing experience. So read this book slowly. A chapter a day is more than fast enough. Maybe a chapter a week would be better. Maybe you want to spend a week rereading the same chapter every day so it sinks into your mind, and so you have time to do the assignments, create the visions boards, and spend time writing in your journal at the end of each chapter. You can choose to rush through this book, or you can choose to take your time and see your new life manifest step-by-step. If you choose to rush, you may see little or no difference in your life. I trust you are reading this book because you know a better life is awaiting you. I know that thought can be scary, but just read slowly, do the exercises, and think about what you read. Pace yourself and as you see yourself making progress, you will see your fear replaced with excitement as your *FITNEVISION* becomes your reality!

Just remember: The journey is the destination! You never arrive. Life is constant and never-ending learning. I call this process: C.A.N.E.L. (Constant And Never-Ending Learning).

When you make it your goal to focus on C.A.N.E.L., your life becomes very exciting. When you're open to learning, growing, and creating, you will meet a lot of interesting people and see a lot of new places because you will be attracting new things into your life. Using the power of C.A.N.E.L. every day, you can't help but grow into a better functioning human being.

I congratulate you in advance for reading this book. Just the fact that you chose to read *FITNEVISION* tells me that you are on the right path to wanting more, and most importantly, to creating your best life ever! I hope you never stop reading, learning, and growing. *FITNEVISION* is just one of many tools from which to learn.

When I explain to people what *FITNEVISION* is, I like to use the metaphor of baking a cake. When you bake a cake, it usually requires more than one ingredient. It is a combination of many different ingredients and flavors that make that one creation sensational. The same is true with *FITNEVISION*. *FITNEVISION* is one of the many ingredients you can add to your journey of mental and physical fitness and personal growth. When we try to learn and grow, I have found that we never get all the answers in one place. We need to have a constant hunger for learning new ways that will teach us better and better how to become our healthiest selves. When you have all different kinds of ingredients, you can bake several different cakes. When you have learned several different strategies for having a healthier and happier life, you will always have tools to pull you out of situations you're not happy about, such as not being healthy or fit, or knowing when to leave a relationship that isn't working.

Being overweight, out of shape, and staying in a negative relationship can cause you to put on more weight and stress you out. This behavior will ultimately release fat hormones that create fat around your gut. The term "spare tire" is used to refer to that layer of fat around the gut. That fat is stress-induced by a hormone called cortisol.

Stress is notorious for secreting cortisol into the body that will actually make you fat.

FITNEVISION is not just about picking up a set of dumbbells or getting on a treadmill—it's a whole lifestyle program. It's mental and physical fitness. But it all starts with your vision of how you see yourself!

FITNEVISION is not just about becoming fit—it's about creating a masterpiece from the inside out called YOU! Becoming your best self inside and out is about being open to the opportunities that will support your health by allowing you to grow into the divine human being you are supposed to be.

I like to think of *FITNEVISION* as having your very own Aladdin's Lamp. You can have whatever you want in your life if you just choose to take action on your visions through the use of vision boards. When you see your vision on a daily basis, you start to take the necessary four action steps toward becoming your vision:

THE *FITNEVISION* STRATEGY:

1. SEE IT! Create the vision.

2. BELIEVE IT! Believe in the vision.

3. SEIZE IT! Take action to make the vision become your reality.

4. BECOME IT! Believe and act on the vision until you succeed and embody the vision.

Using *FITNEVISION* will help you to carry through on all these steps to achieving your vision.

Here's how it works. The mind creates a thought. The thought is then turned into a vision. The action you take is what creates your reality, based on that vision. With the use of *FITNEVISION*, we take it one step further by creating a vision board so you can look at that vision on a daily basis.

Creating a vision and becoming that vision takes time, so I encourage you to take your time in reading this book. Do all of the recommended homework assignments. If you're going to do this program, do it all the way. Get the most out of creating and living your *FITNEVISION* in every area of your life. After all, it is your life, so I say live it to the fullest and with PASSION!

Welcome to *FITNEVISION*. You are about to change your visions, which will change your life!

SEE IT! BELIEVE IT! SEIZE IT! BECOME IT!

Have fun with this book. When you have finished reading it and are implementing the changes recommended, I would love to hear from you about how *FITNEVISION* has changed you!

Sandi Berger

Chicago, Illinois
February 1, 2012

PART 1: SEE IT! BELIEVE IT! SEIZE IT! BECOME IT!

1: *FITNEVISION*: BODY AND MIND FITNESS

FITNEVISION is the combination of mental and physical fitness through visualization. I want to make everyone aware of this power that we all possess. This power inside all of us, which I call *FITNEVISION*, is our own "Mind Theatre" of visualizations. Our minds are always thinking, and when our minds are thinking, they are creating visuals of those thoughts. We are always visualizing; we are just not always aware of this visual energy that we exude on a daily basis.

Keep in mind that when the mind thinks, it thinks in pictures or images, and it is always creating a mind movie. Subconsciously, we choose which mind images or visions we will act out in our reality. We also can make a conscious decision to take action on our visions, such as visualizing ourselves eating healthy foods and exercising. Then we make a conscious choice to take action on that vision.

The driving force behind *FITNEVISION* is to be able to: SEE IT! BELIEVE IT! SEIZE IT! BECOME IT!

Whether it is in regard to fitness, relationships, wealth, or spirituality, we are always creating our lifestyles with visions.

I have written *FITNEVISION* for the sole purpose of creating awareness of the visions that never stop being created in our heads. If you don't like what you're experiencing in life, change the vision! It's that easy—and it's that powerful! It only takes four steps: SEE IT! BELIEVE IT! SEIZE IT! BECOME IT!

1. SEE IT: First, you have to be able to see your goal in your mind.

2. BELIEVE IT: Then, you have to believe that your goal can become a reality.

3. SEIZE IT: Next, you seize your goal when you take relentless action toward it.

4. BECOME IT: Finally, your goal is achieved—you are living your accomplished vision or goal.

Our waking thoughts and our dreams can be compared to going to the theatre and watching a live performance of our lives. The stage is in our own heads. I call this ability to visualize our lives as our "Mind Theatre." We can go through our lives witnessing these performances without knowing who the characters are and what is on the Playbill. Or we can be the director and producer of our own show. It's Your Life. The outcome of your life will depend on the images you create and produce in your reality. We create within ourselves characters who will then play out the roles in our lives that we visualize in order for us to create our destinies. What you focus on and visualize in your mind, you will bring into your reality.

Look around at your life right now. Do you like what you are experiencing? Keep in mind that you are the creator of it all. And in order to change it, you have to be willing to take 100 percent responsibility for it.

So let me ask you a few questions—and keep in mind that you have created everything in your life, good or bad.

- Are you living a healthy lifestyle filled with good eating habits, good sleeping habits, and regular exercise?
- Are you happy with your waistline, or is it getting bigger and bigger with each passing year?
- Do you like your job?
- Are you still in love with your spouse or significant other? Or are you still in that relationship out of fear of being alone?
- Do you have enough money in your bank accounts to support you for a year if you lost your job?

Remember, you are the creator of your life, and before any change can be achieved, you have to take 100 percent responsibility for all of your past visions and characters that have cast you into the reality you are experiencing today.

If you answered, "No" to any of these questions, you need to reevaluate your cast of characters and change your visions. How about the character who believes you can continue eating what you want and still maintain a lean physique? Or the character who quietly says, "Don't worry about your savings account; you're gonna win the lottery!"

Don't buy into the lies. Get in touch with your inner characters and change the cast. These characters are the voices in your head, but they all take on lives of their own inside of YOU!

FITNEVISION is about discovering your inner characters who match those visions and voices.

It starts with your philosophy of life. What is philosophy? It is a set of rules and beliefs that we construct in our minds and act out in the real world. Our visions and our inner voices are the constructs of our living reality. We then assign a character to that particular voice we play out in our conscious state, which becomes our reality.

Taking this concept one step further, if your philosophy is to maintain a healthy body image but you are overweight and have health issues, your inner voice and character are not in sync with your own philosophy. Your belief will not match your performance. This contradiction will cause you to feel frustrated and irritated. We feel frustrated when we cannot achieve our desired results. But how do you fix this problem?

You need to go back and review your philosophy and your visions about being healthy. Change that inner voice and the character will change; then before you know it, your behaviors will start to match your performance. When belief and performance are in balance, the outcome will be positive.

You are always creating your future by the pictures you think and create in your mind and then act out in the real world.

Earl Nightingale said it best: "You become what you think about." As you think, your mind is already creating a visual outcome. It sees your thoughts. If you want to create deliberately to obtain the life you want, you need to:

- Have consistency and awareness of a particular vision.
- Believe in your particular vision.
- Seize your vision and take action steps to make it manifest.

- Allow your vision to become your reality.

FITNEVISION is what happens when your mental vision is brought into physical form. *FITNEVISION* happens when your mental visions spring into action, creating your dreams so they manifest into the physical.

Whether your vision is to be healthy, strong, and fit; to have a loving relationship; to acquire more wealth in your life; etc., you can only succeed when you create from the inside out! That is what *FITNEVISION* is all about.

There is no right or wrong vision. Your visions are like wishes. It's your desired wish that you are commanding in a visionary form. That wish or vision can be anything you want.

Your mind is like your very own Aladdin's Lamp. Every time you challenge your mind with a commanding thought and vision, you are commanding a wish or a vision of what you want to see happen in your life. Awareness and consistency will make those visions come true. You will create the exact characters within you to fulfill your thoughts and visions.

If you don't like what your Aladdin's Lamp is presenting to you, change the vision in your mind. Remember, you are the director and producer of your mind theatre called *FITNEVISION*.

FITNEVISION = FIT MIND + FIT BODY for a
FIT LIFESTYLE

We all operate out of a visionary state all the time. We just don't realize it. The first step for using *FITNEVISION* is awareness. We think about 60,000 thoughts a day, so isn't it time you start to get in touch with some of your thinking and use it to create the life you desire?

Take a look at your life. Everything in your life began first with a thought and then a vision. Now that you have been made aware of the *FITNEVISION* tool, you can use this visionary power to change anything in your life. This visionary power is the ultimate control over one's life. You have always possessed Aladdin's Lamp, and now taking control of your visionary power means realizing that you are the Genie in your life. When you rub Aladdin's Lamp, a Genie appears (that's you); you make a wish (vision), and you make it come true.

The real secret to making wishes come true is through consistent visionary work and taking action on your visions.

Once you have a wish (vision), the next step is to create a vision board around that thought. Look at your vision board everyday and let the Law of Attraction work its magic. What's the Law of Attraction? It's an ancient secret that has been rediscovered in recent years. It basically says that when we want something, and we are open to receiving it, the Universe will deliver it for you. When we don't get what we want, it's because we don't believe it will come. When we believe it, we will see it. Because if you really, really want it, you will make it happen!

Anything we can BE, DO, or HAVE begins with a thought. That thought is immediately transformed into a vision in our mind. That vision is what we act out in our world. Which character is going to play out this vision? Our characters can be the part of our mind that decides to be healthier or wealthier or more loving. Once we decide on the characters, we proceed by taking action on the visions in our minds.

Here is how it breaks down:

SEE IT! (visual) is the Aladdin's Lamp.

BELIEVE IT! (belief) is the Genie.

SEIZE IT! (action) is the actual steps taken toward your visions.

BECOME IT! (vision becomes reality) is your wish becoming true.

SEE IT! BELIEVE IT! SEIZE IT! BECOME IT!

So what would you like to change in your life?

- Are you overweight and out of shape?
- Would you like to be making more money?
- Maybe you want a significant other, or a different one?

Whatever you want, all you need to do is:

SEE IT! BELIEVE IT! SEIZE IT! BECOME IT!

It's that easy!

In the chapters that follow, we will work on how you can learn to achieve anything you want in your life. So let's get started! To start the *FITNEVISION* project, you will need to do the following:

- Read each chapter. Use the blank pages at the end of each chapter to do your homework assignments, create vision boards, and journal your thoughts.
- Keep in mind that when you handwrite your dreams, goals, and feelings in a journal, that journal holds within its writings a very powerful energy that will help you to fulfill your visions and to create awesome vision boards.

- Make a list of 100 things for which you are grateful. This is a MUST DO assignment. You might want to have a notebook or journal on hand for longer assignments.

- Make a list of 100 affirmations that you can refer to as needed. They should be a part of your emotional toolbox. Affirmations are positive things you can say about yourself. Here are a few examples: "I am smart, clever, and witty. I am fun to be around. I am very good at my job. I am capable of making my dreams come true." Make your affirmations detailed and appropriate for your situation. Remember, they all have to be positive. No negativity allowed! We'll use and discuss these in more detail as we work together through this book.

- Make a list in your journal of 100 goals you want to accomplish within your lifetime. Once you accomplish them all, you can just recreate another list. Let's hope you keep making goal lists.

- Have at least one dozen small poster boards on hand in case you want to do larger vision boards. Collect also some glue sticks (for gluing your visions on your board), scissors, and plenty of magazines to find images so you can start creating your vision boards. Feel free to use actual photographs too. Anything that will enhance your vision board is welcome.

Have fun with each assignment and all the vision boards you create for your *FITNEVISION* future.

FITNEVISION HOMEWORK ASSIGNMENT

Do not go on to the next chapter until you have successfully written your three lists.

List One - 100 things for which you are grateful:

_____
_____
_____
_____
_____
_____
_____
_____
_____
_____
_____
_____
_____
_____
_____
_____
_____
_____
_____
_____
_____
_____

List Two - 100 Affirmations:

List Three - 100 Goals before your die:

JOURNAL

Write in your journal how you feel about beginning the *FITNEVISION* journey. Are you excited, scared, resistant, unsure, hopeful?

_____
_____
_____
_____
_____
_____
_____
_____
_____
_____
_____
_____
_____
_____
_____
_____
_____
_____

Keep in mind that when you're green you are growing, but when you are ripe, you are rotting.
~ Author Unknown

JOURNAL

VISION BOARD

Create a vision board using the materials above that you collected to represent what you would like your life to be like. Let your imagination go wild and depict anything you think you would like in your life.

You can use the space below to create a mini vision board or use poster board and go all out!

2: KEEPING A JOURNAL

Something happens to a thought when you write it down. Keeping a journal is a way to keep track of your thoughts and visualizations. Thoughts are pictures in the mind.

You can also keep track of your current goals in your journal. Your journal is for your eyes only. Don't share it with anyone. When you share your dreams and goals with others, you open yourself up to hearing others' opinions, which can diminish your sense of accomplishing your goals. It can be like letting air out of your car tires. You can lose your drive to achieve. That's why whom you hang out with and share thoughts with is so important. Our brains are like sponges and absorb negative and positive energy. Unfortunately, we tend to believe the negative feedback more easily than the positive. That is why your journal should be your sacred space for writing down your dreams, goals, and visualizations.

You can also make your journal your vision book. I have several journals where I cut out pictures from magazines with key words that help me form a picture of how I would like the outcome of a particular goal to look.

FITNEVISION HOMEWORK ASSIGNMENT

Start a journal if you don't have one. It doesn't have to be anything fancy. Buy a spiral notebook with paper and start writing. You can write in your journal any time of day, but the best time to write in your journal is before bed. It's also good to keep your journal in your nightstand right by your bed. When you write before bed, you take those visions and goals with you into your dream state, which can really make them come alive. Your subconscious will keep working out what you want and dream about while you sleep. Keeping those ideas in your dreams by focusing on them before you sleep can help your goals arrive into your reality sooner. Having your journal at your bedside will make it easier if you wake up and have a terrific idea or a thought you want to remember in the morning because you can quickly write it down, go back to sleep, and have it there to benefit you tomorrow.

What you feed your mind before you go to bed makes a big difference—the last thing you watch or read at night you take into your dream state—so focus on the positive. I recommend not watching the news before bed because it is full of negativity and can create feelings of anxiety in you. Instead, write in your journal and then fall asleep dreaming about what direction you want to take your life. It can all start with writing in your journal.

JOURNAL

Write in your journal how you feel about beginning the *FITNEVISION* journey.

_____
_____
_____
_____
_____
_____
_____
_____
_____
_____
_____
_____
_____
_____
_____

What we continually think about eventually will manifest in our lives.

~ Sidney Madwed

JOURNAL

VISION BOARD

In the space below or on a poster board, create an image that represents you journaling and what you will learn and create in your life by writing down your visions, dreams, and goals.

VISION BOARD

3: HOW YOUR VISIONS AFFECT OTHERS

Have you ever heard the saying, "You become what you think about?" Not only is that statement true, but as a result of our thoughts, who we become also has a direct influence on others.

Remember the movie *It's a Wonderful Life?* George Bailey, played by Jimmy Stewart, got to see how his life affected the people in the town of Bedford Falls. He hated his life in Bedford Falls. So Clarence, George's guardian angel, allowed George to see what the lives of the people he knew would have been like if he had never lived. With Clarence's help, George was able to see the impact he had on others, and he learned how important he was in his hometown to everyone. What a gift he was given to see how his life had positively affected others.

When we create visions in our life and are passionate about those visions, we bring them to us or manifest them into our current life. In essence, those visions that then become our reality have an effect on everyone in our life. Even strangers. When you feel good inside and out, you start to smile and that smile will affect everyone who comes into your personal space.

When we envision ourselves as being healthy, fit, and alive with enthusiasm, we start to take steps toward that vision of a person who is healthy, fit, and alive with enthusiasm from the inside out. When we passionately want something and do not doubt that we can have it, the changes that start to manifest in our lives may be so very slight that we don't see them at first. But once you set a passionate intention, it can take on a life of its own. If you passionately want that intention to become your reality, it is amazing how the body and mind start to create it. For instance, if you are serious about cutting back on sugars and fats in your daily diet, don't be surprised if you automatically start adding a little less cream and sugar to your coffee. Before long, you will be drinking your coffee black and enjoying the real flavor—allowing yourself really to taste the true coffee bean in its best form…brewed in a cup!

When you start taking little action steps toward your intention, you give off a certain type of energy. You feel more alive and energized! When you exude this energy, people will feel it and want it. And, of course, some may not want it. When you are around a person who is alive with energy, that energy becomes contagious and will attract people of a like mindset. By the same token, things could go the other way where some people may actually distance themselves from you because they don't want to be around such a high energy person—you might feel like a threat to the less happy life with which they are comfortable—if that's the case, let those people go. You don't need their negativity in your life. You can't win everyone over or fix anyone, but you can feel fortunate that your infectious and passionate energy not only benefits you, but it may also inspire others to become healthier and more optimistic.

Visions are also based on the philosophies we have about our own lives.

What do I mean by a philosophy? We each have a personal philosophy that is our own set of rules, guidelines, beliefs, and concepts that we live by. For example, my philosophy centered on good health means getting the right amount of sleep, putting high quality nutritious foods in my body, and of course, daily exercise. These processes comprise my philosophy for what makes me my best self. And it works for me! I am living proof.

We all do visionary work and set our own philosophies even if we don't realize it, thus creating a vision unconsciously. Instead, what we want to do is to be disciplined and take some quiet time to sit and journal to get in touch with our beliefs. When you take time to write down what you believe, you become more conscious of your beliefs. Then you can decide which of your beliefs is working in your life and which ones have overstayed their welcome. Get rid of what you have believed that you realize is not true and of any beliefs that are holding you back from what you truly want in your life. Then tweak or create a new philosophy that will help you toward your new goals for yourself.

Think of your life up to this point. At some time in your past, you created a vision of how you wanted your life to be and you acted on it. You may have decided to go to college, or you may have decided you wanted a spouse, and then you took action. Even if you didn't think of these decisions as visions to fulfill, that's exactly what you did. You focused on a vision and it showed up in your life. Just look around and you will see your visionary work. Your work will show up in your waistline, your bank account, your business or the type of job you have, your friends, and in your intimate relationships. These are all indicators of visions that you created at some point. These are your philosophies that you live out every day of your life.

If you're not happy with your life, change your visions and philosophies. Then you will have changed your life. Guaranteed!

Here is the formula for *FITNEVISION*:

Vision + Philosophy + Passion + Action = Life Changes

(V+P+P+A=LC)

Let's take *FITNEVISION* to the opposite extreme. If your vision of yourself is as a criminal who steals from others, think of all the people who will be victimized as a result of your vision as a crook. The effect of one injustice done to an individual has an effect on not only the person victimized but also his or her family and friends.

Take Bernie Madoff as an example. In case anyone is not familiar with Bernie's work, he was at the helm of one of the biggest Ponzi schemes in the world. He stole millions of dollars from wealthy people, some even well-known celebrities, by convincing them that he would invest their money so they would get great returns. Through lies and deception, Bernie Madoff manipulated many people to give him money, including elderly and retired people. Because Madoff's situation finally exploded and all these people realized their money was gone, many of these retired people had to go back to work since they had lost their life savings and retirement funds by trusting Mr. Madoff.

HOW YOUR VISIONS AFFECT OTHERS

What a mastermind Bernie was! There is someone who used his visions in the wrong way!

Bernie had a vision and acted on it. Unfortunately, it wasn't the right vision. Not only is he in jail today for acting on his vision, but his criminal act led to his son's suicide and created a life of hell for his wife.

Keep your visions upbeat and healthy. CHOOSE YOUR VERBIAGE WISELY. Words have a huge impact on our lives. We become the words we speak and the visions we create. Speak and think positively and your visions will manifest in desirable and amazing ways for you.

FITNEVISION HOMEWORK ASSIGNMENT

Focus on the words you use. Catch and stop yourself from using negative words. Replace them with positive and uplifting ones.

JOURNAL

Write in your journal about what you realize after you spend some time paying attention to the words you use. Which words do you need to eliminate from your vocabulary, what words can you replace them with? How do certain words—both positive and negative ones—make you feel?

_____
_____
_____
_____
_____
_____
_____
_____
_____
_____
_____
_____
_____
_____
_____

Whatever you assume to be true will become real for you.
~ Dr. Robert Anthony

JOURNAL

VISION BOARD

Create a vision board of how you can influence others for the better.

VISION BOARD

4: LIVING LIFE WITH PASSION

When you live with passion, your life feels and looks very different. When I discovered the true meaning of living my life with passion, I chose to change my inner vision, and then everything in my world changed. So when you change how you see people, those people will change. Only, it won't really be the people who have changed—it's you!

Having that understanding has helped me with a lot of my relationships. This awareness of how my vision determines my outside world has created a feeling of lightness in my inner being, and I became a happier person on the inside. I felt free. I was able to let my true self be exposed because I understood myself and others. Now I no longer take anything personally. Whatever anyone says or thinks about me is none of my business. It's never really personal. It's about how the other person is viewing his or her reality of people. With this knowledge, I started to become really interested in other people and I started to like them.

It is fascinating to me how others think and why some people do what they do. When I meet someone on the street and I smile or hold a door open for him, if it's not reciprocated with a smile or a kind word, but instead, I get a scowl, I just look at that person with compassion, and I wonder what must be going on inside of him to make him so cold. Often, I will then try to joke with those people who won't even crack a smile. Sometimes, I am successful and I get a chuckle or a downright laugh out of them—just maybe that sets the tone to change that particular person's day. We all have a purpose on this planet, and part of my purpose is to make a difference in the lives of others. A big part of that difference is just to put people in a better mood and help them to change their visions. What is your purpose?

My passion for living has taken me on many visual journeys. I have come to appreciate what is happening around me and to feel a deep compassion for people all over the world. Just this morning, I was changing my linens and thinking about how I really love the print on my bed sheets. I then started to think about all the people who were involved in the creation of my bed sheets. First, there's the person who had the vision for the type of pattern to print on the sheets; just by taking action on his vision, *voila!* My bed sheets were created. Then, I thought of all the other people involved in the creation of those sheets and getting them into my hands. There is the manufacturer of the sheets, and the salespeople, and the person who delivers the sheets to the retail store, and store personnel who put them on the sales floor, and finally, there is the consumer—me—who purchases them. If just one of all those people had not taken his or her action step, I would be sleeping on different sheets.

Being passionate is visualizing with gusto. Living in gratitude will keep you in a state of passion, compassion, wonderment, and excitement. When you're grateful for everything in your life, you can't help but be passionate about everything and feel a host of other terrific feelings. The ability to be a passionate person is the ability to look beyond the surface to see what truly is, and with much added feeling and emotion. Everything we do is based on emotion.

I am up and out of the house quite early most mornings because a lot of my clients like to do their fitness workouts before work. I pass by many bus stops where there are hoards of people waiting for the bus to bring them to their jobs. I usually look at the people's faces standing at those bus stops, especially on a Monday morning. I see a lot of faces of sadness. Those people are exuding negative energy while waiting for a bus that will take them to a place they don't want to go to do a job they don't like. Even their one passionate thought, "I can't wait until Friday" is a lot of passionate energy used negatively. That is not the kind of passion you want to possess.

If you are in a job you don't like, or you feel stuck in a body you're not happy with—change it. If you are in a relationship that is giving you more pain than joy—leave it. Or try changing the way you look at those areas of your life, and you may be surprised by how those situations will change. Either way, life is way too short for you to be living a miserable existence. Start your journey toward living life to its fullest by showing loads of gratitude, emotion, and appreciation for everything around you. Search for the good even in the things that make you unhappy. If you have a job you dislike, feel gratitude that it provides you with an income until you find a job you can be passionate. Life truly is precious and can be taken from us in a "nano" second. Every day we live on this planet that we do not experience a passion for living, we are stopping up our creative juices and losing our zest for life. That leaves us not living but being like the living dead, like zombies just going through the motions.

Whenever you feel that zest for life ebbing, it's time to pull out your gratitude list and your list of 100 goals. If you're not excited about your life and where you're headed, change your life in this moment. Get passionate about living, and live an exceptional and outstanding life!

Be a part of the living, not a part of the dead.

FITNEVISION is about looking beyond. Going from GOOD to GREAT, from GREAT to EXCELLENT, and finally from EXCELLENT to OUTSTANDING so we STAND OUT among the rest. We are all capable of being outstanding, passionate human beings. Very few of us, however, are truly outstanding except for the really passionate people. The person who is looking always to improve and continue his or her journey of self-discovery is most likely a person who lives with passion.

FITNEVISION HOMEWORK ASSIGNMENT

Write out your purpose and memorize it! Start to put your purpose into action if you haven't already. Remember, we are all here on this earth for a purpose.

JOURNAL

Journal your thoughts about what you have learned from this chapter. What would it take for you to feel OUTSTANDING? Write about how it feels. Write about how your vision of the world would change if you were passionate about the world around you and you changed your vision of how you saw other people.

_____
_____
_____
_____
_____
_____
_____
_____
_____
_____
_____
_____
_____
_____

You must begin to think of yourself as becoming the person you want to be.
~ David Viscott

JOURNAL

VISION BOARD

Create a vision board of you being OUTSTANDING! Then put that vision into ACTION!

5: CREATING YOUR EMOTIONAL TOOLBOX

This is going to be short and simple. Pull out your journal and create three lists. I asked you to make these lists in Chapter 1. Some of you may have decided to read on and not do them, but I want you to know I'm serious about those lists. They are so important I'm giving you the opportunity to do them again. If you did them already, take the time to make new ones. Now that some time has passed since you made the first set of lists, you may have a new perspective and your lists may have changed. It will be interesting to compare lists and see how your vision has grown and changed already as a result of your becoming conscious of your vision and seeking to have passionate energy.

Here are the lists you need to make to feel and live your vision and passion:

List One: Goals: Write out 100 goals you want to achieve. They can be big or small goals. The important thing is that you write them down. As you achieve each goal, put a line through it. When you have all 100 goals achieved, make another list of 100.

List Two, Gratitude: Write down 100 things you are grateful for in your life! Feel free to go beyond 100. If you created this list earlier, see how your list has changed now. Have you thought of more things for which to be grateful? Make a new list and then compare it to your old one. Always be updating this list. Every day, we can find new things to be grateful for if we keep our minds open to it.

List Three, Affirmations: Create a list of 100 affirmations that will help you reach a state of "blissipline". Affirmations are positive things you tell yourself, such as "I can achieve any goal I put my mind to," or "I attract healthy people to me because I am kind and caring."

"Blissipline" is a word that sets the tone for living in a state of bliss. But in order to be constantly blissful, we need to discipline ourselves regularly to review our list of affirmations and our gratitude list. These lists should be read daily so they become a part of our speech.

Once those lists are ingrained in your thoughts, you will be amazed to watch the person you will become. Remember: We become our thoughts!

You've got work to do. As Nike would say: Just Do It!

FITNEVISION HOMEWORK ASSIGNMENT

Create your three lists. I'm deadly serious that you need to do them.

JOURNAL

Now that you know the word "blissipline", what can you do to achieve "blissipline" in your life?

What have you learned from creating your three lists? Have you learned anything by doing this exercise a second time?

Journal about these questions or any other thoughts you're having about this process.

___

Destiny is not a matter of chance, it's a matter of choice: it is not a thing to be waited for, it is a thing to be achieved.
~ William Jennings Bryan

JOURNAL

VISION BOARD

Create a vision board of what blissipline would look like in your life.

6: BEING UNIQUE

What does being unique look like to you?

Being unique is about being outstanding, about standing out from the rest of the crowd. It means you do things differently. You think and act outside of the box.

Uniqueness is what gets us further ahead in life.

Create a unique way of expressing yourself. How about through your style of dress? Go for different.

One unique way I express myself is through interior design. I am passionate about decorating my home. Ask anyone who really knows me. I like to re-create my home every five to eight years. One thing I hate is having a matching sofa, loveseat, and end tables with matching lamps. I say, "BORING!"

My house is fun, friendly, and very modern, with a lot of unique stuff. Just as an example, I have a white leather coffee table with a smoked glass tabletop. Little leather wedges that serve as seats tuck neatly underneath the coffee table to provide a great tabletop fireplace. It's so great for entertaining. People love it because it is cozy and intimate. I can serve appetizers and cocktails and people can sit and not have to stand at my cocktail parties. It is especially fun when I have a fire going in the tabletop fireplace. That was a great and unique invention. I commend the person who first had the vision to create it.

Guess whose house my friends want to party at, especially on a cold winter evening? Mine, of course. That's because my home is unique, and because I love having people over.

People are attracted to unique. We all learn from each other, so when you stand out from the crowd, people admire that trait and gravitate toward you because you have or are something they want to have or be.

I say stand out in the crowd. Be uniquely you.

If getting that kind of attention makes you nervous and fearful, then it's all the more reason why you should do it.

Challenge yourself. It's the challenges that we overcome that raise our self-esteem and make us stronger emotionally.

Don't wish for something to be over just because it challenges you. Just wish to be better at handling it.

FITNEVISION HOMEWORK ASSIGNMENT

Do one thing that makes you feel or look unique. Create the idea and act on it. *FITNEVISION* it!

JOURNAL

Write about how you can be unique, or what being unique would feel like to you. Write about your vision.

_____
_____
_____
_____
_____
_____
_____
_____
_____
_____
_____
_____
_____
_____
_____
_____
_____
_____
_____

You have to "be" before you can "do" and you have to "do" before you can "have."
~ Dr. Robert Anthony

JOURNAL

VISION BOARD

Visualize your unique self and/or create a unique idea that you can implement in your life.

7: THE YIN AND THE YANG INSIDE

When creating your *FITNEVISION*, feel free to mix it up. What do I mean? If having bicep muscles that bulge a bit with a nice six-pack abdominal section appeals to you—and you're a woman—don't let others judge you by saying, "You look like a man." Gender is an illusion anyway. Yes, hormones separate the genders, but for the most part, we are a mix of both masculine and feminine energies. Do you know a sensitive man? Do you know an assertive woman? I know I do. And no, neither one is gay! It is perfectly okay to possess both of those qualities…and to be gay as well. As a matter of fact, all of those qualities can be sexy.

Let's say for instance that you want to achieve a six-pack abdominal section, whether you're a man or a woman. You can find photos of men and woman who have six-packs. Then make sure you look at the photo of the person with the six-pack daily. What we see in our minds, we bring into our reality! The idea is to imprint in your mind a firm six-pack midsection for yourself. First a thought, then a vision, and then take ACTION!

We're all made up of both male and female energies. I say, if you're a man, tap into that female energy. Find something you can get emotional about. Do it in private if that's more comfortable for you, but do it! Maybe it's a movie that moves you to a wet eye or thinking about a past love. Whatever it is, take twenty minutes to sit quietly and bring out that female energy within you.

If you're a woman, let the male energies out as well. Think of a situation where you may have wished you were a little more assertive. If you can go back and reassert yourself, do it. It may be difficult to do, but do it anyway. You will walk away empowered and feeling in charge of your life. Try it! If you can't come up with a way to assert your male energy, keep it in the front of your mind so that when an opportunity presents itself, you are prepared to move forward and assert yourself. This experience will make you a stronger woman.

Keep in mind that being assertive is different from being aggressive. Aggression is usually done with an anger component. Assertion is a gentler, kinder way of asking for what you want.

Balance is the key in life. We need to balance our Yin and our Yang to feel fully alive.

Gender is an illusion. We are all human beings with blood, guts, and emotion!

To live a fulfilled life, you need to feel all of your emotional powers. I personally love the unique balance that I have between my yin and my yang. I find that balance makes me feel very powerful and empowered.

FITNEVISION HOMEWORK ASSIGNMENT

Take thirty minutes to sit quietly where you will not be disturbed. Visualize your polar opposite. What would he or she look like? How would your yin or your yang dress? How would his or her emotions be expressed? Really, really get into it.

Women, let those male energies flow through you and feel them. Assert yourself wherever you can.

If you're a man and some emotion comes up for you, go ahead and cry, cry, cry. Contrary to what Frankie Valli sings, Big Girls and Big Boys DO Cry! It's called being a HUMAN!

Talk to both sides of yourself. Give your yin and your yang a name. See them and incorporate them into your life. Embracing that other side of yourself may just be what you need to get into the best physical shape of your life!

JOURNAL

Write in your journal about your male and female energies. Especially focus on those energies from the opposite gender. How can you bring about more balance between them to benefit you?

_____
_____
_____
_____
_____
_____
_____
_____
_____
_____
_____
_____
_____
_____
_____
_____
_____
_____
_____

If you correct your mind, the rest of your life will fall into place.
~ Lao Tzu

JOURNAL

VISION BOARD

Create a vision of yourself with your yin and your yang, your male and female energies, all aspects of yourself balanced.

8: DANCING

Dancing is an expression of your inner emotion transferred to your feet. Movement to music creates a sense of freedom. Freedom to express whatever it is you are feeling in any given moment. I love to dance. Anyone who knows me knows how passionate I feel about dancing.

Sometimes when I dance, I am moved to tears, and at other times, to a place of euphoria. Dancing can be very intense for me. It's my anti-depressant drug of choice.

You don't have to qualify to be on *Dancing with the Stars* to enjoy dancing. Dancing is about freedom. The freedom to move freely no matter what it looks like. It's your expression of energy moving through you and around you, allowing you to express who you are, how you feel, what you want and desire, what is your vision for yourself.

If you're not a person who likes to dance, I recommend dancing in the privacy of your own home so you don't have to deal with feelings of self-consciousness, embarrassment, or intimidation by others who may be on a dance floor in a public place.

In your home, you can put on your favorite music and just move around any way your body chooses. It doesn't matter what you look like when you dance because you are in your home so nobody can see you. If you have a family and want to dance alone, wait until nobody is home and then put on your favorite music, your dancing shoes, and get crazy with the freedom of movement. Dancing freely will release stress, create good brain chemistry for you, and you may even feel euphoric. Try it! You'll like it.

Try dancing on a day when you may be feeling blue. Create an opportunity to put on your favorite music and just dance. Just let the music flow through you and then move to it. It is a wonderful feeling to have the freedom of movement.

When you become comfortable in your own skin while dancing, invite others to join you and share the energy of moving freely.

Sometimes you have a locked emotion that you can't put into words. By dancing, you release feelings that may help you better express the locked emotion you may be feeling.

You don't need a reason to dance. Just dance!

FITNEVISION HOMEWORK ASSIGNMENT

Part 1: Dance Dance Dance!!

Part 2: Dance some more.

Part 3: Dance with family and friends.

JOURNAL

How do you feel when you dance? Write about dancing or any other thoughts you have about creating your vision and freedom for yourself.

___

Taking time to relax my mind and body is as important to my success as working on my goals.
~ Richard Carlson, Ph.D.

JOURNAL

VISION BOARD

Create an image of yourself feeling free.

9: WHAT IS YOUR PURPOSE FOR BEING ON THIS PLANET?

Have you ever taken the time really to think about why you were placed on the earth?

If not, now is the time to give this topic some serious thought. Maybe you are here to teach, to help a special child, to create a special song that the world will be singing, or maybe just to be an inspiration to others. Think about why you are here. We are all here for a reason, and we have been given various assignments to complete before we go back to our original form…which is dust.

Without getting too metaphysical on you, I just want you to think about your purpose for your life.

My purpose is quite simple. It is three things. Here they are:

1. Make a difference in the lives of others no matter what age I am or they are.

2. Have fun and always look for the humor.

3. Make money so I can afford to continue growing and learning. I like living a quality lifestyle too. With money,

I can do the activities that will help me to grow, and ultimately, to help others.

I love learning from others and I love teaching others what I have learned. That is my purpose. Now it's time to think about yours.

FITNEVISION HOMEWORK ASSIGNMENT

Think about your purpose for being here. Write it down in your journal. Review it daily so it becomes a part of you and your life.

JOURNAL

Write about your purpose in life. What parts of it are you fulfilling? In what areas do you need to do more to fulfill your purpose, and how can you fulfill it?

___
___
___
___
___
___
___
___
___
___
___
___
___
___
___
___
___
___

The most important thing with any goal is you first have to believe it is possible!
~ Sandi Berger

WHAT IS YOUR PURPOSE FOR BEING ON THIS PLANET?

JOURNAL

VISION BOARD

Create a visual image of you and your life purpose.

10: BIRDS OF A FEATHER USUALLY SHARE A SIMILAR VISION

Have you ever heard the saying, "You become whom you hang around with"? Or how about, "Lay down with dogs and wake up with fleas"?

My point here is that you have to be very selective with whom you associate on a regular basis. We are all like human sponges, so if you are spending your precious moments on this planet with people who are going down a path of negative energy, I say, "RUN!" If you don't, that negative energy will be absorbed into your psyche until you start to act out from that same energy. Don't think you can influence negative people with your positive energy. Unfortunately, the people who carry negative attitudes and energy always win out. You will absorb their negativity before they take on any of your positive energy.

Nothing is more important than feeling good all the time. If you find that you are slipping into a negative space, find a reason to feel good. Pull out your gratitude list. Always reach for a better thought. Have a list of good thoughts in your journal so you will always have instant access to better thinking. It's important that you find a better thought that will create a better vision for you; then you will gravitate toward that vision and take action.

But if you are trying to create a better thought and vision and you are surrounded by negative people, that vision will soon turn sour. How can you tell when you have absorbed others' negative energies and visions? By how you feel. If you lack energy and feel lethargic—BINGO! You have just caught someone else's negativity, just like you would catch a cold from someone else. This time it's the negative energy germ you've caught.

Pull out your lists of affirmations, your gratitude list, and your goals, and change your thoughts as soon as you can. This one action step will change your negative thoughts into positive ones. This change will then create a vision of positive energy that will change your life!

Keep in mind that if you feel a negative emotion and it's not from someone else's influence, you are resisting something you want. You will quickly feel the toll this resistance will have on your body, and ultimately, it could cause you to stop pursuing your visions by slowing down your daily activities. In time, such resistance will affect your health, both physically and mentally.

When you find yourself feeling negative and you realize it's because of resistance, perhaps caused by fear of failure or fear of success, the best thing to do is to "Let Go."

To "Let Go" means to let go of your worries, anxieties, and fears. To realize you cannot control everything, and to trust that you, being your best self, will be enough to make everything work out for the best. Replace those fears with wonderful thoughts and visions of yourself as succeeding and watch how your body responds. Rather than envision failure, envision yourself succeeding. Let go of fear and you will be surprised by how quickly things will fall into place for you.

FITNEVISION HOMEWORK ASSIGNMENT

1. Make a list of the people who have a negative impact on your life. Make the decision to limit your time with these people.

2. Make a list of ideas for how you can meet positive uplifting people.

JOURNAL

What do you need to do to limit the negative people in your life and replace them with positive and uplifting people who will share or support you in your vision?

___

As a man thinks in his heart, so is he.
~ Proverbs 23:7

JOURNAL

VISION BOARD

Create a vision of the type of people you want in your life.

11: GOAL SETTING IS PART OF CREATING YOUR *FITNEVISION*

Pick one thing you want to achieve in your life. Make it a goal. Write it down in your journal.

1. What is the goal? Be specific and definite.

2. Write the target date you would like to achieve it.

3. List the action steps you are going to take.

4. Create a vision board for your goal. Cut out lots of pictures and key words that will enhance your internal fire for achieving that goal. Get excited and enthusiastic when creating your vision board. Make your board as big as you would like, maybe even poster size so your vision sits on an easel for you to look at every single day.

5. Look at your vision board every day and take one action step per day until you achieve your goal.

6. Write about your vision and the steps to reach it in your journal.

This one exercise can be done for everything you want to accomplish in your life, whether it is fitness, health, more money, better relationships, etc. You can do many, many vision boards, one or more for each one of your goals. You can even make small vision cards using index cards with affirmations pertaining to your specific goal. Carry them with you so you can refer to them frequently.

Creating a vision board is truly a pathway to achieving your best self ever!

Goals are dreams with wings, especially when they are written down in your journal.

There is a real body-mind connection to goal setting when your goals are actually written down.

Do not use your computer to create your journal or to write. Actually use a pen and paper to write out your goals. Writing by hand creates a higher frequency of energy for achieving your specific dreams.

When I wanted to manifest my sports car, I wrote in my journal about how I would feel in a black BMW Z4. Then I cut out a picture of a BMW Z4 and put my face in the driver's seat. I actually cut my face from an old picture of myself and glued it right in the driver's seat of the picture. I placed this picture on the front of my refrigerator so I could look at it daily. Now, can you guess what happened?

My picture became a reality! The most exciting day was the day I drove off the lot in my brand new 2007 BMW Z4. Yee Haw!

You too can make your dreams come true with the power of *FITNEVISION!*

FITNEVISION HOMEWORK ASSIGNMENT

Pick the one most important goal to you right now and focus on ways you can achieve it, using the steps above.

JOURNAL

Write about the goal you want to achieve. How does it feel? How will you make that goal, which is currently a dream, become a reality for you?

(At the bottom of the page you'll notice there is a quotation like always, but this time, and for some of the quotations in other chapters, I want you to insert your name and I want you to repeat these sayings until they become your mantra. Go ahead—say them out loud to yourself until you come to embody these thoughts.)

_____
_____
_____
_____
_____
_____
_____
_____
_____
_____
_____
_____

I take action today on my dreams!
~ (insert your name here)

GOAL SETTING IS PART OF CREATING YOUR *FITNEVISION*

JOURNAL

VISION BOARD

Create a vision board around your goal.

12: FAKE IT AND WATCH YOURSELF MAKE IT

Have you ever heard the saying, "Fake It Till You Make It"?

The point is that when you act as if—you "fake it"—that something you want has already happened, you attract that something into your life so it becomes true. Here's how it works:

First, I want you to create a vision in your mind of your perfect life. Be outrageous and over the top. Let your mind run wild. Then start to collect pictures that resemble your new up and coming life! You guessed it…slap 'em on a vision board with some great positive words that match the vision.

This can be really fun if you can let yourself go.

So, for instance, you want a perfect body. Even though we know there is no such thing, imagine what your perfect body would look like.

What about the perfect career? Or maybe you want to have a business of your own? Explore in your mind what that would look like and feel like.

Imagine that money is not an issue in your life. What does that look like and feel like?

Your relationships are so inspiring and healthy. Feel that vision.

Imagine your sex life being phenomenal with a person you absolutely love and adore.

Create a huge vision board with all of these visions and look at it daily. Be creative with color and borders. Make it your masterpiece!

I created a vision exercise mat. First, I created my visions on two big pieces of poster board by taping them together as one. After I pasted all of my vision pictures and affirmative sayings and key words on the poster boards, I scanned the vision board and had an exercise mat made through a company called Yogamatic.com

You can do the same thing. Now every time I do my workouts on my mat, I see my visualizations.

I love looking at my visions every day. They make up my roadmap for my life.

When those visions are all accomplished, I will create another exercise mat and start the process again. Remember, the destination is the journey and the journey never ends. We just keep growing if we allow ourselves to make that choice.

Study your visions by looking at them every day. Create another vision board as needed with new visions and study it daily.

I have always dreamed of becoming an author on the subject of living a healthy lifestyle. My vision mat has visions of this happening, and *voila*! Here I am today writing my book!

You will become what you think about and vision about. Make sure you have the right roadmap of visions in your mind and you will be excited about your life. Guaranteed!

FITNEVISION HOMEWORK ASSIGNMENT

Make a list of every area of your life you want to make better so you are sure to include all your visions for yourself on the giant vision board you are now going to make, per the chapter you just read.

JOURNAL

Journal about all the visions on your vision board. Why did you include them and how will you feel when they are achieved?

_____
_____
_____
_____
_____
_____
_____
_____
_____
_____
_____
_____
_____
_____
_____
_____

I create my best life vision and manifest it!
~ (insert your name here)

JOURNAL

VISION BOARD

Create your vision board with all the areas of your life represented that you listed above.

13: ONE CHOICE AWAY FROM A FABULOUS LIFE

Think about it—we are only one choice away....

We are only one choice away from having better relationships.

We are only one choice away from improving our eating habits.

We are only one choice away from creating a better self-image.

We are only one choice away from making more money.

We are only one choice away from feeling sensational.

We are only one choice away from making our dream lives one choice away!

You get the idea!

You choose daily how your life is going to be. You are one choice away from making better choices and creating better visions. Remember every choice is a vision. Take action on improving your visions, and then make choices to create those visions in every area of your life.

Maybe this is the day you decide to get a membership to a health club. Or this could be the day you start exercising by taking that first walk on your lunch break.

When you make a choice, you are taking charge of your life, good or bad, depending on the choice. If the choice today is to get started exercising, and you proceed to take action, I guarantee you will feel terrific, first because you're taking action toward your goal, and within a few days, you will physically feel better as well. All because you made a choice and took action.

Maybe this is the day you decide to leave an abusive relationship, and as a result, you open yourself up to meeting healthier people. All because you made a choice.

Maybe this is the day you decide to eat better. You start to feel better and look better. All because you made a choice.

The word choice is only five letters long, but the action that word represents has a huge impact on how we choose to live our lives every single day.

Just recently, I had to make a choice regarding my home. I listed it with a well known realtor. I have often said, "If Bonnie the Realtor can't sell it, nobody can!" But as we all know, the real estate market is in the toilet these days. Nevertheless, I really wanted to sell my condo, and buy a condo in a more upscale part of Chicago.

Despite all of my effort, and the efforts of a very good realtor, we could not even get a breakeven price. So I had to make a choice to take my condo off the market. I made the decision that for the next three to five years, I will wait until the market changes.

After my realtor removed my home from the multiple listing service, I felt disappointed, so I immediately created a vision of how my place would look with brand new furniture. I pictured exactly the type of furniture, wall hangings, and colors on the walls I wanted. I put together a vision board with pictures that I took off the Internet and ideas of contemporary modern furnishings. Now, I have always loved leather, and white leather is incredibly sharp if done tastefully.

To make a long story short, I just recently had delivered my Italian white leather sofa. My friends thought I was crazy to get leather since I have a dog that could scratch it up. But I followed my heart and vision board, and now my pooch and I are very comfy cozy in our newly furnished condo. I didn't let other people's thoughts or opinions about what kind of furniture I should have stand in my way.

I know I will now be happy to be in my home for the next several years.

Trust your own decisions and choices. And when needed, create a vision board and take action!

The CHOICE is yours!

FITNEVISION HOMEWORK ASSIGNMENT

Make yourself aware of all the choices you are making and start a list of those choices that have not worked in your favor. Write the choices that haven't worked for you on a piece of paper and then burn them.

Start immediately replacing those old choices with healthier ones.

Get in touch with how you're feeling about your choices. If you find yourself rationalizing one of your choices, you have not made a wise choice. You have to feel 100 percent positive about your choices.

JOURNAL

Journal about the choices you have made, healthy and unhealthy, and what you can do to replace the ones that aren't healthy.

_____
_____
_____
_____
_____
_____
_____
_____
_____
_____
_____
_____
_____
_____
_____
_____

Fit people create fit pictures over and over in their minds. You will always act on the pictures you create.

~ Sandi Berger

JOURNAL

VISION BOARD

Create a vision board around a choice you need or want to make.

: **VISION BOARD**

14: TRUST IN FAITH AND MAZEL

I trust that faith and *mazel* are working on my side.

In Yiddish, *mazel* means "luck."

There is a saying in Yiddish: You have to have a little mazel with the hard work.

If one of my goals takes a U-Turn, I will just reconfigure my steps and once again apply faith and mazel to learn from any mistakes I have made and to get back on my roadmap to success. I always trust that I am on the right track; there is no right or wrong when taking action toward a specific goal—only learning and growing, and an occasional readjustment. By the Law of Attraction, I attract the right things I need to help me achieve my goals. And so will you!

Focusing on your goals and believing in mazel, however, doesn't mean that you set a goal to do a vision board and when finished, you just sit around and wait for your goal to be magically achieved. No! You have to work at your goals every day.

I start each morning with a cup of coffee, light a fire in my tabletop fireplace, make sure my phone is off, and sit in silence. I let whatever needs to come up in my thoughts rise to the surface; then I let go of those thoughts—any worries or fears—and replace them with faith and trust. Many of my best ideas and goals for creating my *FITNEVISION* life have come to me during this time I call my morning coffee meditation.

After this process, I write in my journal any new ideas, goals, or other thoughts I believe will be important to help me fulfill my ultimate destiny of being healthy.

I have created so many fitness routines and exercises as a result of this time I give myself every morning.

Find your uninterrupted time just to think! Watch how mazel will work in your life if you let it! Have FAITH in you!

Find your place and the time of day where you can either meditate or just sit in silent contemplation for at least 20-30 minutes. Write about whatever comes to your mind in your journal.

Then do one thing daily toward achieving your goals.

FITNEVISION HOMEWORK ASSIGNMENT

Create your silent time. Since you're probably new to this assignment, think about and write down 100 things you would like to achieve before your die. If you did this assignment earlier, do it again to see how your list has changed. I suspect your vision and goals have gotten bigger and better.

Work toward achieving every one of those goals on your list. Having so many wonderful goals will give you something to contemplate in your silent time and work on in your free time.

If you find that you have accomplished all of your goals on your list before your time is up, congratulations! Now it's time to create a new list.

Always keep reaching for more and keep those visions coming.

JOURNAL

Write down your thoughts following your daily meditation time.

_____
_____
_____
_____
_____
_____
_____
_____
_____
_____
_____
_____
_____
_____
_____
_____
_____
_____
_____

If you change the way you look at things, the things you look at will change.
~ Dr. Wayne Dyer

JOURNAL

VISION BOARD

Create a vision board of as many of the 100 things you want to achieve before you die that you can fit on it.

15: IF YOU DON'T LIKE YOU, NO ONE ELSE WILL

I want you to look at yourself in the mirror. Really look into the mirror and really look at you. Stare into your eyes. Look at the color, texture, and length of your hair. Look at your skin, your pores, your skin tone. Now check out your ears, your mouth, your cheekbones, and your chin. Really explore your face. For some, paying this much attention to yourself may be hard to do. But if you can't give yourself direct eye contact, how can you expect to have eye contact with others? Even if it's hard, just do it anyway. That's how we work through our fears—by facing them and neutralizing the intensity of what we feel fearful about. Next, I want you to take a good look at your hands, the length of your fingers, and your fingernails. Do you like your hands? Check out your arms. I know a lot of women think they have flabby upper arms. If you're one of those women, say, "So what?" That's just who you are right now. And you can change it!

Continue this mirror exercise by inspecting your entire body. Get to know your body.

When you have completed this mirror exercise, pull out your journal and write five things you absolutely love about your body; it could be anything from your fingernails to your head.

Next, list five things you love about you, such as your sense of humor, your style of dress, or maybe you like that you are a very compassionate person. Whatever those things are, write them down. It's important to list at least five things. Why five? Because it's too easy to find one or two things you like about yourself. Listing five pushes you really to look at yourself inside and out. I'm sure you can find five good things about yourself. Go ahead and find them! Appreciate yourself!

After you have discovered the ten things you love about yourself, from the inside out, notice how you feel. Notice how your internal vision of yourself changes. Maybe your face has softened and you are able to smile. Maybe you just let go of some labored breathing and let out a heavy sigh. Or maybe you just feel elated.

Now, list two things you dislike about yourself. I say two because I don't want what you dislike to be your focus. Remember, what we focus on we bring into our reality. After you have written the two things you dislike about yourself, notice your internal visual. How do you feel now? I bet you're a little more hunched over, feeling low, and you have lost some of your energy to perform at your best today.

Take those two things on your list that you dislike about yourself and turn them into likes. For instance:

Dislike: I don't like my hair. It's too dull.

Change to a Like: I would love my hair with highlights. (Then take action and go get highlights.)

Dislike: I dislike the way I respond when people say, "Good morning" to me.

Change to a Like: Say "Good morning" to five people every day. If they say, "Good morning" first, it doesn't count. Take action and start saying, "Good morning" with a big smile and thank God for another day to be alive. Watch how your mood may change little by little to a better feeling.

This process of changing our dislikes to things we like about ourselves is very important. In order to create visions for a better quality of life, you have to believe in yourself. Part of believing in yourself is liking yourself!

When you have a belief in your abilities, your resulting performance will show you how much your feelings are like a barometer for whether or not you are believing in yourself. That barometer of how you are feeling is an indicator that tells you how well you are doing in working toward your goal.

Your performance should match your beliefs to get the best results. If it doesn't, change your belief or your performance level.

For me, my performance relates to writing this book. I believe this book can be an asset to a lot of people, so I really want to finish it and get it published before the end of the year. My performance level is kicked into high gear because I believe I can get this book done by the deadline I have set for myself.

If I were just lollygagging and taking my sweet time writing, then my performance would not be matching or reflecting my belief. Therefore, I would be out of balance, and that would cause conflict in my mind. This conflict would show up in my body, probably in the form of lowered energy and feeling like I don't want to do anything.

FITNEVISION is 99.9 percent thought. And thoughts become pictures in your mind. You become what you think, picture, and envision on a daily basis. Those thoughts and pictures create your beliefs and performance levels.

Change your thoughts and the pictures in your mind will change; that will change your belief and your performance level, which will ultimately change your life.

You are holding the remote control. If you don't like what you see on the screen…change it!

Understanding this segment is what it means to take 100 percent responsibility for your life. Only you have the power to create your life. Inside and out!

FITNEVISION HOMEWORK ASSIGNMENT

Get in touch with your most dominant thought or vision, which is a belief you hold about yourself.

JOURNAL

Write about how well your performance level matches your greatest belief about yourself?

Picture your vision on a sixty-inch flat T.V. screen. If you don't like what you see, imagine yourself picking up the remote control and changing the screen. Now what do you believe? How is this going to change your performance around that thought or belief?

_____
_____
_____
_____
_____
_____
_____
_____
_____
_____
_____
_____
_____
_____

I let go of old habitual, self-defeating thoughts.
~ Richard Carlson

JOURNAL

VISION BOARD

See the picture of your thought/belief. How does it look?

Create an image of the dominant positive thought or belief you hold about yourself and how you want to perform in regards to that belief.

16: F.E.A.R. AND OTHER LIES WE TELL OURSELVES

Ninety-nine percent of what we fear never happens to us. Here is a great acronym for the word fear.

F – False

E – Expectations

A – Appearing

R – Real

I didn't create this acronym, but whoever did was right on!

What happens to the majority of people who set a New Year's resolution to lose weight and get into shape? They never follow through. They may start their resolution, but five days later, it's a "has been." One of the many definitions of success is commitment to consistency.

When January 1st comes around, the gyms and health clubs are packed, but by January 5th, the gyms and health clubs are practically empty again. Statistics show that any given health club can oversell its memberships by 60 percent. Why? Because health clubs know that most people will pay high membership fees and monthly dues, but they will never use the facility for which they are paying. If every member showed up at the same time at a given health club, you wouldn't be able to move. It would be wall-to-wall people. In all my years of working out and training, I have never run into that problem.

My belief is that most people, while they might complain about being out of shape, are really quite comfortable with where they are at. The real problem is that most people live from a fear-based place in their heads. They let fear get in the way of being their best selves ever! So, what are these people afraid of? Looking and feeling good?! You can get very comfortable feeling bad about yourself. Here's how you can tell whether you are one of those comfortable people. If you are constantly complaining about how you look and feel, and you believe that you really want to be healthier, what are you doing to change it? How would you rate your performance level based on your belief that you want to be healthier and in better shape? Your performance will give you your results. If you are not satisfied with your results, you have two choices:

You can step up to the plate and improve your performance level, meaning you will get serious about your belief, or

You can change your belief to match your performance.

You see, just because you have a belief, it doesn't necessarily mean you want to do anything about it. This imbalance will cause conflict in your mind, which diminishes your energy so you end up doing nothing but complaining. This situation is all a form of resistance, which is another form of fear. Keep in mind that resistance and fear come in many disguises. Your real aim is to recognize those masked intruders, refuse to let them be in charge, and change the situation so your performance and results are satisfactory to you.

I will use myself as an example. When I am embarking on something new that is exciting and good for me, I start to develop an irritated or sour stomach. This problem ends up being a convenient distraction from my goal because I become focused on how to get rid of my stomach irritation. It takes my attention away from what I want to accomplish. Or I may go into a fit of sneezing when I start to take action on a belief—another form of resistance. Our minds are very tricky. We have to be on high alert twenty-four hours a day so we don't let our fears and our subconscious take control. Even our dreams can show us signs of resistance.

For a long time, I did not realize that these minor health ailments were forms of resistance and fear.

Then one day, it finally hit me! I can be my own worst enemy and sabotage my personal growth and well-being. Even writing this book at this moment is creating that sensation in my stomach. But now I have learned just to ignore that little devil known as resistance because he does not want me to succeed. And believe it or not, when I ignore him, the stomach irritation passes and I can plow through any project I am currently undertaking and accomplish my goals. However, remember, this devilish energy of resistance that we all possess from time to time does not like to be ignored, so it will be persistent. Just be aware of it, and then say out loud, "Resistance, you will not prevent me from losing weight and getting in shape (or whatever other goal you have). You may win some small battles that go unnoticed, but the war is ultimately mine to win!"

We all have that little devil called Resistance that is working against us. The trick is to find that evil energy that lurks in our minds, and that ultimately destroys our success, and just ignore it and persevere.

Awareness is key. Once you are aware of this pesky resistant monster, you are in control to stop it!

FITNEVISION HOMEWORK ASSIGNMENT

Make a list of the areas of your life where you may be resisting or fearing good coming to you. For each item on your list, ask yourself: Why am I resisting it?

JOURNAL

Write about the most significant area of your life where you are feeling resistance. Why are you resisting and how can you overcome that resistance?

_____
_____
_____
_____
_____
_____
_____
_____
_____
_____
_____
_____
_____
_____
_____
_____
_____
_____
_____

My mind is capable of much more than just worrying.
~ (insert your name here)

JOURNAL

VISION BOARD

Empower yourself by creating a vision board or illustration of you overcoming or defeating your personal resistance monster.

17: C.A.N.E.L. (CONSTANT AND NEVER-ENDING LEARNING)

If you are at a place in your life where every day you are operating out of habit or you are on auto pilot, you are in what I call a "visual slump!" Snap out of it now! Start to program yourself to wake up every morning feeling like today is going to be an adventure. And then it will! What you focus on, you bring into your reality.

Each morning when you wake, ask yourself, "What new thing am I going to learn and act on today that will enhance my future?"

Maybe your new thing will be a new exercise class or a new food that you have wanted to try but you haven't yet. Or better yet, maybe you will learn a new tool for how to handle a stressful situation in your life. When you are stressed, you usually just want the stress to pass. Instead of wishing the stress were over, wish you were better at handling such situations. Learn a new tool.

Meditation is a great tool to have in your emotional toolbox. Here's a great visual: Picture yourself going to your emotional toolbox and pulling out the meditation tool. What does your meditation tool look like? Visualize it.

WOW! How powerful and empowering would that be?

C.A.N.E.L. stands for: Constant And Never-Ending Learning. If you apply the C.A.N.E.L. method to your life, you will start to create and learn new skills to keep you challenged. Apply the C.A.N.E.L. method everyday and watch what happens in your life—you may be pleasantly surprised.

The definition of a human being is a person who is just being. HOW BORING!!!

When we are learning and doing and creating, we are happiest. Therefore, instead of being human beings, we should aspire to be "human doings."

In order to be a happy, healthy "human doing," we need constantly to be learning and growing. Hence, C.A.N.E.L.—Constant And Never-Ending Learning.

In order to have an exciting, challenging, adventuresome life, you need to keep reinventing yourself. How do you do that? By using the C.A.N.E.L. method.

Pick a topic that you would like to learn about. Maybe you would like to learn more about a certain artist. Just start the process of C.A.N.E.L. You can start at the library by taking out a book and reading about your new topic or endeavor. Create a vision board right in your journal for your new goal.

C.A.N.E.L. is not just about fitness—it's a whole package of constant learning and creating that human doing called YOU! When you are learning and growing, you are creating a healthier, happier YOU! That creation will spill into you wanting to feel and look better about yourself. It's all connected. Keep challenging yourself with new material.

Another way to keep learning is to Google it! Whatever it is… Google it! I can't begin to tell you how Google has given me so much learning power. Just the Internet, in and of itself, is a plethora of learning. It's never-ending.

There is a saying, "When you're green, you are growing, and when you're ripe, you are rotting." Never, never be ripe. Always stay green and live the C.A.N.E.L. way of life.

FITNEVISION HOMEWORK ASSIGNMENT

Create a list of your C.A.N.E.L. goals.

C.A.N.E.L. (CONSTANT AND NEVER-ENDING LEARNING)

JOURNAL

Write about your C.A.N.E.L. goals and the skills you will acquire from what you learn.

___

Keep in mind that when you're green you are growing, but when you are ripe, you are rotting.
~ Author Unknown

JOURNAL

VISION BOARD

Create a vision board for each new skill or piece of information you will learn by using the C.A.N.E.L. method.

VISION BOARD

18: GETTING IN TOUCH WITH YOUR CAST OF CHARACTERS

We are all made up of many different characters. Let me ask you this: Do you feel like you're the same person around all people? Sometimes, don't you feel more aggressive around certain people, or maybe you are more likely to take charge around other people? At other times, maybe you feel on the defensive, or more vulnerable, or maybe even intimidated around other types of people. We play different character roles daily, depending on the situation and the people we are around. We all play different characters, even if we are not always aware of it.

I find Donald Trump to be quite a fascinating personality, but I know if I had the opportunity to sit down and talk with him, I probably would feel a little intimidated being in his presence. That would be my "Intimidated" character. I don't like playing that character, so in order for me to diffuse those intimidated feelings, I would visualize myself having a conversation with Donald Trump where I felt the way I want to feel in his presence—perhaps confident, or simply enjoying myself. I could play another of my characters—"Humorous"—who would know how to get Mr. Trump to laugh or at least crack a smile. Of course, I am only visualizing the scenario as I would like it to happen, but remember, we get what we visualize and focus on!

By pre-visualizing the outcome first (See it! Believe it! Seize it! Become it!) and by playing out exactly how I would like that meeting with Donald Trump to be, I would be taking on the role of my Confidence character. Now, when the day comes that I do have the opportunity to meet Donald Trump (I say that with a "Fake it till you make it" attitude), I will most likely feel more confident in Mr. Trump's presence—because I have already been in that situation in my mind.

One of my all time favorite celebrities is Jennifer Aniston. She is someone who is really an inspiration to me. Her authenticity comes through loud and clear. Being in her presence would be like being with a best friend. I look forward to meeting Jennifer one day. I believe it will happen. Why? Because I have focused on it and have rehearsed meeting Jennifer in my mind through my visualizations. The character I believe I would be in her presence would be my "Authentic-Relaxed-Accepted" character. See it! Believe it! Seize it! Become it! That's the power of visualization. We all possess that strength.

If you want something badly enough, you can bring it to you. That's how powerful our minds are. That's the power of visualization.

We can BE, DO, or HAVE what we want simply by seeing it first in our minds and believing it! So, be careful what you think about most of the time. You may wake up one morning

GETTING IN TOUCH WITH YOUR CAST OF CHARACTERS

and find it right in your backyard—good or bad! You decide. Your life is exactly the way you create it!

I will use Donald Trump one more time as an example.

Donald Trump had a laser-like vision to build skyscrapers, and *voila!* I think there is a skyscraper in most major cities called Trump Tower! Just think…it all began with a thought!

Jennifer Aniston had a vision of being an actress. I don't think she envisioned the magnitude of success she has achieved, but she certainly has achieved her vision and much more!

So if we don't like any of our little characters that show up from time to time, change them in advance. Create a vision of how you would like to be in a given situation. Do a vision board around your vision. Rehearse it in your mind until it is not even a vision anymore because it has become your reality. Pick a character you want to be in a situation, practice being it, and *voila!* You become it. We become what we think about all the time.

Keep in mind that life can catch you off guard. There may be a time when you don't feel prepared to play a situation a certain way. With this awareness, I say be prepared to be prepared at a moment's notice. Have your characters dressed and ready to go whenever they are needed. It's like you're the understudy in waiting for that role. And when you find a situation you're not prepared for, if you take a second to remember you are a character playing a role, you'll find yourself giving a convincing performance that will then turn your character-acting into the reality you want.

All you have to do is visualize how you would like to be in a particular situation. Create the character in your mind and start visualizing yourself as that new character. With practice, character role-playing will get easier, and it will even become a lot of fun—I promise.

GETTING IN TOUCH WITH YOUR CAST OF CHARACTERS   143

FITNEVISION HOMEWORK ASSIGNMENT

First, make a list of all your characters that you recognize you have played out at one time or another. For instance:

- The confident character
- The heartfelt, compassionate character
- The PMS-ing, irritable, bitchy character
- The generous, supportive character
- The insecure character
- The angry character
- The happy character
- The sad character
- The having a good hair day character
- The "I feel good today" character
- The assertive character
- The aggressive character
- The ego-maniac character

You get the idea. Add to your list any characters I haven't covered. The list could be endless.

Now remember all these characters are a way to look at feelings and emotions. I have labeled those feelings as characters. As Shakespeare said, "All the world's a stage" and your life is a never-ending performance.

Get in touch with your characters. We all have them.

Now that you have your cast, let's create the stage. Pick a situation that is coming up in your life. It might be a review with your boss, or a blind date, or better yet, a party you plan to attend where you really won't know a lot of the people there. Choose the character you want to play in a given situation. Visualize how your character will carry him- or herself in that situation. How do you want to play the character you will be in that situation?

Or you can replay a situation where you wish you had acted differently. Recreate the character you would like to have been in that situation. Practice visualizing the character you would like to be in that situation.

JOURNAL

Write about how you will feel playing a character in a future situation or a past situation you want to improve. What will you say, how will you feel, what will be the result?

_____
_____
_____
_____
_____
_____
_____
_____
_____
_____
_____
_____
_____
_____

We all have a champion within. Discover yours.
~ Sandi Berger

JOURNAL

VISION BOARD

Choose a situation and the character you want to be in that situation and create a vision of it.

VISION BOARD

19: CHANGE WHAT YOU SEE AND YOU CHANGE WHAT YOU GET

Your mind is always thinking; therefore, you're always creating visions in your mind, whether you realize it or not. Remember, the mind thinks in pictures. How you see yourself and your life is exactly what you have manifested in your life right now. Look around you, and if you don't like what you see, change it!

If you want things in your life to change, you are going to have to change things in your life.

Since this book is about creating your lifestyle and fitness vision, how are you seeing your body image? How about your life image? If you're happy with what you see, then you are on the right track.

If you're not happy with your lifestyle and your body image, then what are you willing to give up in order to improve them?

You can't keep doing the same things over and over again and expect diffcrent results. In order to create change, you must re-evaluate what you are currently doing and make conscious changes.

For instance, if you are eating three healthy meals a day, but they are huge in portions, maybe you need to adjust to five smaller, healthier meals a day. This change may jumpstart your metabolism to achieve a better result for your body image.

If you're going to the gym and doing the same workout day after day, you need to reassess your exercise program and change it up to give your body a shock. Your body may then respond with more of the results you're trying to achieve. That one change could make a world of difference in changing your body image. Also, keep in mind how resistance may be playing a key role in whether you are seeing the change you want. Our minds are very clever, so they often will disguise resistance, as I discussed previously.

You see, what we focus on we manifest. Most people aren't even aware of what they are consistently focusing on and visualizing on a daily basis. They know they are not happy, but they can't seem to get a handle on why they aren't feeling truly happy in their lives. It's all dependent on what their visions are and where they place their focus.

FITNEVISION HOMEWORK ASSIGNMENT

Make a list of everything you want in your life that you currently don't have. Then look for the places where you are resisting it. Look deep and hard because, remember, our minds like to trick us into rationalizing why we can't have something we want, simply because change can be scary.

JOURNAL

How are you currently visualizing your life and your body image?

If you like what you see, write about it.

If you don't like what you see, write about how you feel because you don't like it. Feel free to get all your frustrations out on the page. Don't forget to include any forms of resistance you may be feeling.

Then write about what changes you are willing to make in order to achieve your body image and lifestyle goals.

_____

_____

_____

_____

_____

_____

_____

_____

_____

_____

_____

_____

Your brain and your body are permanent. Changing how you think and your body shape isn't!
~ Author Unknown

JOURNAL

VISION BOARD

Create a vision of your life as you would like it to be one year from now, free from resistance of all the good things you desire for yourself, your body, your relationships, your health, your entire life.

20: YOU ARE THE ULTIMATE DRIVING MACHINE—INSIDE AND OUT

One of the most exciting days in my life was when I was able to achieve one of my big goals. That was the day I purchased my Z4-BMW—The "Ultimate Driving Machine" as BMW likes to call it.

When I bought my Z4-BMW, I asked my salesman, "What kind of gas should I use in my new 'Ultimate Driving Machine'?" He immediately replied, "Premium car, premium fuel." That was an "Aha!" moment for me. I am always trying to think of clever sayings and slogans that will keep me in a constant state of affirmation. Now whenever I think about what I want to eat, I use the saying, "Premium body, premium fuel." Nothing but the best fuel goes into my body. If I have a day where I am craving something bad, I reach into my toolbox of sayings and slogans for a better craving tool, and I usually select the healthier snack.

The same practice should apply to what you are putting into your mind. I suggest taking thirty minutes for yourself every day to read something positive, whether it's a self-help book or affirmations. For those thirty minutes, fill your brain only with premium thoughts.

Nothing tastes better than looking and feeling your best!

That day when I drove out of the dealership in my brand new BMW-Z4, I was looking and feeling my best! I was the Ultimate Driving Machine inside and out!

FITNEVISION HOMEWORK ASSIGNMENT

Make a list of any positive sayings or slogans you have heard, especially ones that have inspired an "Aha!" moment for you.

JOURNAL

Select some of your positive sayings that created "Aha!" moments for you and write about how you can apply them to your life.

_____
_____
_____
_____
_____
_____
_____
_____
_____
_____
_____
_____
_____
_____
_____

When I change my focus, I change my life.
What I focus on, I bring on.
~ (insert your name here)

JOURNAL

VISION BOARD

Create an image of yourself as the Ultimate Driving Machine, filled only with premium fuel.

21: EAT HEALTHY: WHAT YOU PUT IN YOUR BODY DETERMINES YOUR PERFORMANCE

In my opinion, the key to a happy life is to have good dietary habits. When you saturate your body and your cells with high quality, nutritious foods, it affects everything else in your life. When you're healthy from the inside out, it will lessen irritability, your judgment of others, and in some cases, even your rage. Good nutritious foods help to keep your hormones and weight in balance. You will be happier as a result.

I remember when computers first became a household name and the acronym G.I.G.O. ("garbage in, garbage out") became popular. G.I.G.O. is so very appropriate still for today's fast food bingers. When you put garbage in your body, you are certainly going to get garbage out. If you want your body to perform at its best and highest level, then only put good, healthy foods into it. Happiness is about feeling great both inside and out. So, make the healthy choice when it comes to food.

I'm gonna let you in on a secret. You already know what to do as far as eating habits are concerned.

You know if you are in a McDonald's restaurant, and the cashier asks you, "Do you want a regular size of fries, or do you want to SUPERSIZE your order?" what your answer should be. But just in case, let me help you. Your answer should be, "Neither." Tell the cashier you want the grilled chicken sandwich, no mayo, hold the bun. Start training yourself to order a healthy meal, no matter what type of restaurant or eating establishment you find yourself in.

It just takes practice and common sense. Trust me; we all instinctively know what foods to put in our bodies.

EAT HEALTHY

FITNEVISION HOMEWORK ASSIGNMENT

Go online and find five menus from five of your favorite eating establishments. Print them out. After you have all the menus in front of you, circle with a red pen all of the healthy choices.

Now when you go into a restaurant, you are prepared to make better choices.

JOURNAL

Write about your relationship with food. Why do you make unhealthy choices? What can you do to change that behavior? What is one thing you can do today to make a difference? What good food choices can you make to replace the bad food choices in your life?

_____
_____
_____
_____
_____
_____
_____
_____
_____
_____
_____
_____
_____
_____
_____

What we put into our bodies has a great deal to do with how we look and feel.
~ Sandi Berger

JOURNAL

VISION BOARD

Create a vision board with only healthy pictures of food, like fresh fruits and vegetables. Keep it where you will see it constantly until you begin to crave healthy food.

22: GETTING IN TOUCH WITH YOUR DISOWNED SELF

I have actually made a list of all the people who have made an impact on my life and all the lessons I have learned that have made me the person I am today.

I have had many different kinds of relationships in my life, and I have taken a piece from each and every one of them to create a better me. I am still creating me because I am still learning from others and I know I have many more people to meet in my life who will teach me ways to become my better me.

Here's a perfect example of how I got in touch with a part of me that I shut down. Many, many years ago, I was very quiet and people thought of me as shy. Today, when I tell people that, they will say, "Whhaaatttt? Sandi Berger, shy?" People who didn't know me in my younger days just can't believe I was ever shy.

When I was a lot younger, I used to attract people into my life who were very vocal and could talk to anybody at anytime. I used to feel very intimidated around people with that personality type. Then I began reading self-help books, and in many of the books, I stumbled onto the topic of reclaiming your disowned self. I went to work on that piece of my puzzle, and even though I felt intimidated by outgoing people, I started to copy their behaviors and gestures. It was a little scary practicing these behaviors on others and trying to play the self-confident and outgoing character. It felt so awkward for me because it was so far from who I thought I was at that time in my life. Thanks to author Susan Jeffers, who wrote the wonderful book *Feel the Fear and Do It Anyway*, I followed her directions, and as a result, I plowed through those fears until I took ownership of my disowned self and made my own self whole.

I can't recommend Susan Jeffers' book enough. Even if you have no obvious fears, read *Feel the Fear and Do It Anyway*. You will find it freeing and empowering. I give it a five-star rating.

What is that part of yourself that you disown, or that is better known as your disowned self? Our disowned self is the part of ourselves that we try to bury. Usually, it's a part of ourselves that we don't like or don't want to acknowledge. However, when we don't face that part of ourselves, we usually attract it through an outside force. Usually that outside force will show up in our significant other, or maybe a friend or even a coworker, or possibly, all three. However it shows up, it will keep coming back to haunt us unless we face it head on, surrender to it, accept it, or change it.

The most influential people in my life have been the ones I've dated. These people provided a big learning experience for me because I came to realize that whenever I would pick a potential life partner, I was actually picking a reflection of my own disowned self. For example, I would attract partners who were physically unfit or the antithesis of what I wanted to be. I also would spend my time trying to change that person into being the person I wanted; since you can't change people who don't want to change, this situation was self-defeating. Eventually, I realized what I had to do was focus on what I needed to change about myself. It took me a long time to recognize this truth and make the change, but it was true.

Until we take responsibility for our disowned self and begin to change the situation, we will continue to attract people into our life who will mirror that disowned part of us and who constantly remind us of that part of ourselves. Otherwise, that disowned part of ourselves could very well become the source of irritation in our relationships. The very thing we disown in ourselves is the thing we don't like in our relationships. It's at this juncture that people start to blame others for the deterioration of their relationships. Once you have an understanding of this situation, however, you can take 100 percent responsibility for your life and relationships. When we take responsibility for our feelings in all of our relationships, and we don't burden someone else with our "blame stuff," then we have the making of a healthy, communicative, and very loving relationship.

Now, let's take this one step further. If you are not taking 100 percent responsibility in all of your relationships, and that includes your relationship with your parents and your siblings, you probably are overweight, experiencing pain in your body, or just generally unhappy. Most likely your unhappiness is a manifestation of an internal conflict that has been dismissed or disowned due to a lack of personal responsibility. Here is where personal growth and soul-searching can save your life. Remember, a life unexamined can lead to your being among the living dead! When too many parts of yourself are disowned, your body will manifest its unhappiness in a physical form. It could show up as panic anxiety disorder, depression, chronic fatigue, or a host of many other self-created illnesses. Living your life with these maladies is not how God meant for you to live. Yes, life is hard, but when we face our demons head on, we can live fully alive and with lots of good energy to spread around the planet.

We are all made up of so many different feelings and emotions. Some we let show, and some we try to keep hidden, even from ourselves. It's those hidden feelings that certain relationships bring to the forefront. Those relationships expose our disowned self to us! If we would only take responsibility for ourselves and our disowned parts of ourselves, I bet the divorce rate would go way down in our country.

So what does all of this have to do with health and fitness? Our unhappiness, our disowned selves, and how we manifest that unhappiness in our bodies will impact our physical form in one way or another.

Believe it or not, the pieces of ourselves that we disown are a big part of who we are, and they affect how we will project ourselves both mentally and physically.

If you have a friend who is always going to the gym and eating healthy foods, and you feel threatened by that behavior, you will either find a new friend or jump on that friend's bandwagon. If you choose the latter, you are then coming to terms with your disowned self—the part of you that wants to be fit and healthy. If you choose to find friends who love to eat the wrong foods and think going to a gym is a waste of time and money, then from time to time, you will probably be confronted with a person who lives a healthier lifestyle as a reminder to get into shape. The choice is always yours. You can face your demons or keep running.

As the saying goes, "You can run, but you cannot hide."

It is our disowned self that keeps us overweight and unhealthy. Our disowned self also will present us with resistance to changing our lives into the kind we want.

Remember, resistance has many disguises. Take off the mask and get real with your disowned self!

FITNEVISION HOMEWORK ASSIGNMENT

Sit quietly for thirty minutes and try to recognize what you might be avoiding or disowning.

JOURNAL

Write about the parts of your life that you feel you are disowning. When you get in touch with that piece of yourself, start going to work on changing it and taking responsibility.

Keep writing about your experiences as you go through this process. You may find that once you work through changing one disowned part of yourself, another disowned part of yourself appears. Don't let this stop or frighten you. It's all part of the *FITNEVISION* process to a new and improved you!

Feel the fear and do it anyway.
~ Susan Jeffers

JOURNAL

VISION BOARD

Create an image of your disowned self and you welcoming your disowned self home. How will that reunion feel? Envision your disowned self redeemed, or as a vital and happy part of your full self.

VISION BOARD

23: FALLING IN LOVE WITH YOU

Can you love yourself unconditionally? That would mean accepting yourself, flaws and all. No more calling yourself names like, "idiot, stupid, fat, or ugly." The list of names we call ourselves is virtually endless. In some cases, we call ourselves names so often that it becomes a knee-jerk reaction whenever we fail at something.

Instead, let's look at failure as positive. Have you ever heard the term, "Failing Up"? All that means is that without failure, we will not grow.

From this day forward, start "Failing Up." Make a vow never to talk unkindly to yourself. Start by making a conscious effort that every time you curse at yourself, you will change it right at the onset. So if you catch yourself saying, "I'm such an idiot," change it immediately to "I am a very smart person who just made a booboo, and I will do right the next time." Keep failing up until you don't curse yourself anymore. Start saying, "I love you, _____ (insert your name)." I love you, Sandi Berger!

Take yourself out on a date. Yes, you heard me correctly. Put on one of your favorite outfits and take yourself to your favorite restaurant. After dinner, go to a movie you have been dying to see. For some of you, this exercise could really be stepping out of your comfort zone. You know what I'm going to say to that: "Feel the Fear and Do It Anyway!" When we fear something, we need to go in the opposite direction to conquer that fear. You can't go over or under a fear—you have to go through it in order to heal it.

This exercise alone will help you make the significant changes needed to get on the path to a healthier lifestyle.

When you start to love you, you start to take care of you.

Go ahead. I dare you to take yourself out on a date and fall in love with YOU!

If you do this exercise, I want to hear from you personally and have you tell me about your experience. Email me at: lifebydesignfit@aol.com

FITNEVISION HOMEWORK ASSIGNMENT

Create a list of at least fifty positive words that best describe you.

JOURNAL

Write about the date you went on with yourself, or about all the reasons you like yourself. What do you enjoy about yourself that makes you a person you want to date? Write about anything else that makes you feel good.

_____
_____
_____
_____
_____
_____
_____
_____
_____
_____
_____
_____
_____
_____
_____

Only those who dare to fail greatly will ever achieve greatly.
~ Robert F. Kennedy

JOURNAL

VISION BOARD

Create an image of yourself that embodies the positive thoughts you have about yourself.

24: IN REAL ESTATE, IT'S ALL ABOUT LOCATION, LOCATION, LOCATION.

IN MANAGING A HEALTHY LIFESTYLE, IT'S ALL ABOUT DISCIPLINE, DISCIPLINE, DISCIPLINE.

There is something to be said about discipline. When we are disciplined and follow through on our goals, it just feels so good that it empowers us to set more goals and accomplish them.

For instance, writing this book has taken a certain amount of discipline. When I decided to write this book, I set a goal to spend at least one to two hours per day writing. When I completed that daily goal, my book was complete. Now I feel such a sense of accomplishment. Discipline in itself just feels great!

The same need for discipline applies to fitness and health. When you set a handwritten goal, let's say, to lose ten pounds, you start taking action steps toward achieving your goal. Your goals must be handwritten. When a goal is handwritten (versus, typed on the computer), it has much more energy and impact on actually achieving that particular goal.

You can use the pages in this book to journal, but eventually, you are going to need to purchase an actual notebook specifically for journaling. Just keep in mind that it holds more energy to accomplish a handwritten goal than to have it typed in a blog somewhere on your computer.

After you have set an intention for achieving your goals, you are ready to take ACTION. So if the goal is to lose ten pounds, your action steps might be:

Action Step #1: Join a gym and hire a fitness trainer.

Action Step #2: Learn what your fitness trainer has to tell you about your fitness program and nutrition.

Action Step #3: Put your program into action by eating right and exercising.

Once you take these action steps, you will be on your way to manifesting a healthier lifestyle. After that first session with your new trainer, you will be so excited because you took action, and you are now disciplining yourself to achieve the goal of losing ten pounds. If you should have a bit of a setback, talk to your trainer. If you opted not to have a fitness trainer, then you need to set up a toolbox of ways to overcome a setback. One good tool would be a list of affirmations. A second tool is to focus your vision on the end result. How will you look and feel when your goal is achieved? Picture yourself buying a new outfit that you have wanted. How does that outfit look on you once you weigh ten pounds less?

If your concern is about the cost of a fitness trainer, remember that hiring a professional is not about the cost; it's about the investment in yourself. Aren't you worth it?

Don't forget that all of your goals should be handwritten so they will have a more powerful impact on your thoughts. You can write your goals right in your journal, or get a separate notebook for listing goals only. As you achieve each goal, put a line through it and move on to the next goal.

Once a goal is handwritten and you really want to achieve it, you will magically start to take action steps toward achieving that goal.

FITNEVISION HOMEWORK ASSIGNMENT

Review your list of 100 affirmations and have them on hand to use as part of your toolbox when a setback takes your focus off your goal.

Review your list of 100 goals. When you achieve them make another list.

It's fun drawing lines through each accomplished goal.

Feel the power of discipline with written goals and action steps taken.

JOURNAL

Write about how you can create a disciplined way to achieve your goals. Don't forget that discipline is really "blissipline"—discipline leads to your creating bliss when your goals are achieved.

_____
_____
_____
_____
_____
_____
_____
_____
_____
_____
_____
_____
_____
_____
_____

I make good decisions, and because I do,
I achieve outstanding results!
~ (insert your name here)

JOURNAL

VISION BOARD

Pick the goal you most want to achieve on your list of 100 goals and make a vision board for it that represents the steps you will take to achieve that goal.

25: IT'S NOT JUST FITNESS. IT'S A LIFESTYLE PACKAGE.

How serious are you about being healthy and fit? On a scale of 1-10, how would you rate your seriousness about being fit and healthy? If you said, "five," then you are not convinced that being fit and healthy will increase your quality of life. I suggest then that you create two vision boards. For the first one, I want you to cut out pictures and sayings from magazines that describe you today.

What do you look like? What kinds of things do you tell yourself on a daily basis that you are aware of, such as "I'm fat! Or I hate my thighs," etc. Cut out letters to make those words. Then put the words on your vision board, and try to find pictures to match the words. You get the idea.

On the next vision board, I want you to create how you would like to look and feel.

Once both of those vision boards are completed, take them and lay them side-by-side. Look at the one that depicts the way you look today. Write down your thoughts and feelings in your journal.

Now look at the vision board of where you want to be headed. Write down your thoughts and feelings in your journal.

Put away the vision board of how you look and feel today. Keep out the vision board of how you want to look and feel and place it where you will see it daily. Set a date. Give yourself at least three months. But be realistic.

Day and night, look at the vision board of how you want to look and feel. In three months, or the time you have allotted for your goal to be achieved, pull out your vision board of how you were. You should see a significant change in how you now see yourself.

FITNEVISION HOMEWORK ASSIGNMENT

I'm not kidding about those vision boards. Get started.

JOURNAL

Write about the differences between how you currently see yourself and how you will feel when you become the person you want to be. Write any other thoughts that come to mind that can help you achieve the goal of becoming the person you want to be.

_____
_____
_____
_____
_____
_____
_____
_____
_____
_____
_____
_____
_____
_____

My intuition is my higher self guiding me. I trust and embrace it!

~ (insert your name here)

JOURNAL

VISION BOARD

Create a vision board for the things you tell yourself daily and how you currently feel about yourself.

26: YOU REAP WHAT YOU S.E.W.

S — SLEEP

E — EATING HABITS

W — WORKING OUT

If you are getting at least eight hours of sleep a night, eating five small and healthy meals every day, and sticking to your workouts, you will feel phenomenal. Period, done, the end!

Start today and keep track of your sleep hours. Track the time you go to bed and the time you wake up.

Before you get into bed, make sure your bedroom is dark. Sometimes a streetlight can shine in your bedroom window. Any light in your bedroom at night lowers the melatonin levels in your brain, which can make it hard for you to fall asleep. Also you want to make sure there are no intrusions like a phone or a computer left on. Turn off all electronics before bedtime.

DO NOT watch the news before bed. We are bombarded with many negative topics on our news programs. That is the last thing you want on your mind before a good night's sleep.

Put gentle thoughts into your mind before bed, such as reading your goals and dreams, or reading something uplifting and positive before bedtime.

Keep track of your daily eating habits. Write down what you eat and the time of day. You should be eating at least five small meals a day, roughly one every three hours. At the end of the week, look over your logins for eating, and critique where you can improve, such as drinking more water or having a little less sugar in your diet.

Last, keep a record of your workouts. Write down what you did on a given workout day and the areas where you need to improve. So, if during your last workout, you lifted eight-pound dumbbells for bicep curls and you did a smooth 10-12 reps, lift ten-pound dumbbells today. Keep track in your journal so you can see your progress.

Create sheets for your workouts, eating habits, and sleep. Use an extra journal just for this purpose.

In order to create a wonderful feeling in your body, you have to accept fully and embrace where you are right now.

We tell ourselves so many lies about our bodies that we then choose to believe. Set your goals within reason. Baby steps. If our demands are too high, and we can't make the necessary physical changes to our bodies to meet our high demands, we end up sad, depressed, and overeating. Don't let yourself fall into this cycle. Take control of your mind and your body will follow.

STOP THE MADNESS right now! Get yourself living a healthier lifestyle.

So many people struggle with diet and exercise because they place such high demands on themselves that they end up doing nothing to improve their bodies. The emotional demands people place on themselves create so much anxiety that the possibility of starting a workout program, only to fail, is so huge that most people won't even start an exercise program—they just assume they will fail. But remember, we want to keep "failing up" so we can do it better next time. Failure is success turned inside out!

I have a client who still believes that eating one big meal a day will help her to lose weight. I have tried to explain to her that this eating style will actually cause her to gain weight and lose muscle mass. When you don't put enough food in your body, your metabolic set-point is lowered and will slow down, which will cause weight gain. By eating five small healthy meals every day, you will keep your metabolism stoked so it will continue to work for you rather than against you for the entire day. Think of your metabolism as a fireplace. When you put several pieces of wood on the fire, the fire gets bigger and produces more heat. The same happens when you eat five small meals a day. Your metabolism has to work harder to burn up those meals and actually create heat in your body.

Remember, we reap what we S.E.W.

Did you know that happiness is your natural state of mind? That you have the power to be in a constant state of happiness if you can just get control of your mind and your thoughts?

Our world is as we choose to see it. As you see it, you believe it, and ultimately, you become it! That is what *FITNEVISION* is all about. Creating the fit and healthy lives we imagine for ourselves by turning them into reality.

FITNEVISION HOMEWORK ASSIGNMENT

Make a list for each of the S.E.W. categories of what you need to do to improve in each one:

Sleep	Eating Habits	Working Out

JOURNAL

Write about anything that is keeping you from achieving your S.E.W. goals. What do you need to do to change this situation?

_____
_____
_____
_____
_____
_____
_____
_____
_____
_____
_____
_____
_____
_____
_____

The higher your energy level, the more efficient your body and mind. The more efficient your body and mind, the better you feel to achieve outstanding results in your life.
~ Tony Robbins

JOURNAL

VISION BOARD

Create a vision board that reflects your S.E.W. goals.

27: ACCEPTING YOURSELF RIGHT HERE, RIGHT NOW!

Being in a people-oriented career, I hear so many stories from people about how unhappy and depressed they are. Usually, they are blaming a situation or a specific person for their depression and sadness. Constant sadness.

Folks, keep in mind that when you feel sad, lonely, and depressed, it is no one's fault except your own. You have to accept that you are ultimately the only person responsible for how you feel. If you wish to make progress with this book, you need to accept responsibility for your feelings right here and right now. Now I'm not saying that there won't be times of sadness and pain, or times when someone does something to hurt you or set you back. At those times, you need to feel those feelings, but only to get them out of your system. Don't let yourself stay in that state of mind forever. Be sad or angry for a day and then move on.

But what if you get stuck? You may have some problem or person at this moment that is causing you to be unhappy, so the question you may be asking yourself right now is: "How do I change a thought and move past this situation so I can feel good?"

First, accept where you are in this moment and feel it! Put a time limit on the time you will allow yourself to feel bad. Don't let your thoughts control your life and your emotions. If you're feeling bad on a regular basis, then you're asking yourself the wrong set of questions all the time.

Take back your life by asking yourself better questions. You may be asking yourself, "Why does this always happen to me?" With that kind of question, you are setting yourself up to be the victim, and you know what that feels like—not very good. A better question might be, "How will this situation I am going through make me a better person?" or, "What am I learning from this experience, or what can I learn from this situation?"

When you do feel unhappy about something, don't just wish that you were strong enough to handle it. With constant and continuous practice, you will get through your difficult situation with more ease by asking yourself better and better questions. We all experience feelings of sadness and grief, and we need to feel those feelings. This process that we go through from time to time in life will get a whole lot easier if you are better prepared by asking better questions. Visualize how you want the outcome to be. Write it down in your journal.

Always be thinking of a more empowering question, or create some visuals that will lift you up. For example, you could think about a newborn baby or a warm summer day; maybe you dream about sitting on the beach and enjoying the breeze and the sunshine. How about all the people in your life who love you? Imagine yourself being happy in their presence. One thought I like to have when I'm stuck in this situation is, "If I had never been born, how would my non-existence affect the lives of others?" It's that *It's a Wonderful Life* question again. We all influence and inspire each other in so many ways that we don't think about. Right now, hopefully, I am inspiring you through this book.

What are the conversations you are having with yourself? What do you keep telling yourself over and over that is making you feel bad about yourself? Realize that you are telling yourself a set of habitual lies and buying into them.

I have been told that I live in a fantasyland. Well, with all my goal planning and dream building exercises that I do on a constant and continuous basis, I guess I am in fantasyland, but I'm having the time of my life there!

FITNEVISION HOMEWORK ASSIGNMENT

Make a list of everything in your life that bothers you and who or what you blame for it.

Now look at your list and figure out where you are lying to yourself or being irrational in terms of the blame. What can you do to gain back control of these situations rather than allowing yourself to feel like a victim?

JOURNAL

Is there a person, current situation, or event from your past that you are holding onto that only brings you sadness, anger, or misery? Journal about why you keep holding onto that pain. How would you feel if you let go of that problem? What can you do to move past it? What time limit will you set for yourself to move on?

_____
_____
_____
_____
_____
_____
_____
_____
_____
_____
_____
_____
_____

Every person you meet and continue a relationship with is a mirror of some part of you.
~ Sandi Berger

JOURNAL

VISION BOARD

Create a vision board of yourself in your fantasyland! Let your imagination run wild as you envision what your life can be!

VISION BOARD

28: CONNECTING WITH YOURSELF AND OTHERS

When we are embarking on a *FITNEVISION*, such as weight loss and creating a healthier lifestyle, we must work on having an excellent relationship with ourselves—to the point of really loving ourselves. When we love ourselves, we will do whatever it takes to stay healthy. It's when we fall off the bandwagon that we need to sit ourselves down and say, "What's up? What's going on inside of me that I am giving up on this vision? I love you, _____ (say your full name), too much to let you throw in the towel."

Then pull out the vision board of that particular goal and rethink your vision. Proceed to get up, dust yourself off, and do it again! I don't like to use the word "try." I prefer Nike's slogan: "Just Do It!"

Keep your vision boards and journaling on hand because they are two very important factors for keeping you on track with your goal.

Any goal is a challenge. Family and friends may try to talk you out of your goal. They may say things like, "It's too hard. You'll never make it. You never finish anything you start… blah, blah, blah…." So be careful with whom you share your visions and goals. If you do share them with a naysayer, develop a backup plan for such encounters. Start to develop a confidence in yourself so that, no matter what others think, say, or do, it will not affect your ability to plow straight through to achieving success on your given goal. Remember, you can always cut the conversation short and walk away.

If you find yourself in a situation where people are unsupportive of you, you have two choices: stay or leave. I say, "Get the hell out of there, and go look at your vision boards and read your journal for some positive affirmations."

Here's a quick story about a situation I was confronted with not that long ago. I was getting involved with a network marketing product that I truly believed in. It was a juice made with pure Acai berries and had loads of health benefits. I wanted to get this product out to the world so people could start cleansing and healing their insides with this amazing juice.

One person at a time, I had built quite the team to promote the product. My network marketing business was growing with rapid speed. Being a fitness trainer, I wanted all of my clients to know the benefits of using this product. So I approached one client of mine after four years of training her. I shared with this client all the benefits she could achieve with this product. Her comment to me was, "When you fail at this network marketing business, I will be there for you." WHAT! When I FAIL! I thought to myself, "I cannot continue training this person who is just waiting for me to fail." Can you believe that this person is a psychotherapist to boot? I was appalled. I immediately ended our session that day and our working relationship. You truly become whom you hang out with, whether it is a family member, a friend, a coworker, or even a client. I did not want that negative energy permeating my life.

Make sure you are working on that connection with yourself so you, too, can protect yourself from those Negative Nellies.

Keep yourself out of the path of verbal bullets. Verbal bullets can kill your spirit and destroy your future if you let them.

Remember, you always have a choice. One choice is just to walk away.

FITNEVISION HOMEWORK ASSIGNMENT

Make a list of all your friends whom you believe to be Capital F friends. Capital F friends are those you can trust with anything you choose to share with them.

Next, make a list of the small f friends—those you can't trust. You might decide to let these people remain in your life, but be careful about what you tell them. They are the friends who will probably drop off your radar screen as you get healthier and healthier. That is what happened for me. I have attracted friendships of a quality that far surpass my old chums.

JOURNAL

Think about dreams and goals you have had. Write down what they were and the people who encouraged you and the people who didn't support you. How did you feel about those situations and people? Are those people still in your life?

___

I trust myself and my instincts.
~ (insert your name here)

JOURNAL

VISION BOARD

Ask your Capital F friends to join you in a vision board party. You can all bring magazines, poster board, and anything else you want to use. Share with each other what your visions are, and then help one another find images and words for their vision boards.

VISION BOARD

29: THE WILLS, WON'TS, AND CAN'TS

There are three very different types of people. The ones who *will* achieve their goals. The ones who *won't*. And the ones who *can't*.

What makes the Wills different from the Won'ts and the Can'ts? One word…FEAR!

The Wills usually know that no matter what fears get in their way, they will overcome them and complete the mission. Why do these people always succeed?

Secret: Because they have the ability to keep their eyes on the prize, which is the end result, the actual completion of the goal itself. That is the prize. The reward is the benefit of achieving that goal.

The Wills know how to focus on the end result. They don't let negative self-talk rule their lives! And they don't allow others' negativity to affect them. They usually will just walk away. They also know how to combat that inner voice that is pulling them down and trying to make them quit! They have their toolbox set and ready to go at a moment's notice, and it's all stored in their brains! When the going gets tough, the Wills get going.

The Wills are following their visions of where they want to end up. They can **see** it! They **believe** it! They **seize** it! And then they **become** it! There is no stopping the Wills. They are the people. The Wills have a list of affirmations and a toolbox of strategies that they can resort to when the going gets tough. A Will kind of person has developed these techniques by doing exactly what you are doing now. Reading and learning, and preparing themselves for their futures with love of the self.

Have you ever watched the television show *The Biggest Loser*? This program is composed of Wills, Won'ts, and Can'ts.

The Wills win. The Can'ts end up voted off, and the Won'ts lose some weight, but they give up midstream and lose out as well.

Why is it that some people can lose 400 pounds while others struggle with just losing ten? It's all in the mind, and the mind is the determining factor in everything we do. As we have talked about in the previous chapters, the mind thinks in pictures, and when we create the right pictures or visions, the body follows through with the action steps. But you have to believe that you can do it!

So, if you're a Can't or a Won't, your vision is clearly different from a Will's vision.

Change your vision. Believe in your vision and I promise you will change your life!

FITNEVISION is not just about fitness; it's an adaptation of learning how to create and change your life so you can have a healthy lifestyle every single day you are alive!

FITNEVISION HOMEWORK ASSIGNMENT

1. Create a vision for something in your life that you know you must change but up until now has been one of your Won'ts.

2. Create a vision board around your new vision.

3. Take action immediately on your new vision. Do one action that will bring you closer to accomplishing that vision. When that action is complete, write the next action down in your journal, and take that action.

Action by action taken will get you to the end result, and voila! You will be celebrating your accomplished goal.

Reward yourself with something big when you complete this Won't that you turned into a Will.

JOURNAL

Write about something in your life that used to be a Won't or Can't. How did you feel once it became a Will? What is another Won't or Can't in your life that you want to turn into a Will? How will you feel when your Won't becomes a Will that is a reality?

_____
_____
_____
_____
_____
_____
_____
_____
_____
_____
_____
_____
_____
_____
_____
_____
_____
_____
_____
_____

A loss is a lesson and a win is when you take that loss and grow from it.
~ Author Unknown

JOURNAL

VISION BOARD

Take your Won't or Can't and create a vision board of what it will look like once it becomes a Will.

30: SEE IT! BELIEVE IT! SEIZE IT! BECOME IT!

See it in your mind. Believe it in your heart and soul. Seize it and you become what you envision for yourself. Whether we realize it or not, the mind is always thinking, and it is thinking in pictures. Another way to describe this process is "visual thinking." What do you think dreams are? Visual thinking.

All of us have had the experience of a nightmare from time to time. Do you remember waking up in the middle of your nightmare, scared to death and trying to shake it free? Nightmares are an example of the power of our visions that go on in our heads. We all have a tremendous power right between our ears. We have the power to create visions of how we would like our lives to be and how we would like to have our bodies look and feel, just through conscious and focused visions. Vision boards are what help us to create visions and bring them to reality. And when you look at your vision boards daily, you start to attract to you what you need to create your ultimate vision.

If you make the decision to change your thoughts, your visual thinking, you can go from having negative pictures in your mind to positive pictures in your mind. If you really focus on making this one change, you will be changing the way you think, feel, and ultimately, look. So, in essence, you can think yourself FIT. What the mind thinks and sees, the body will follow by turning into a reality.

A very well known writer and speaker, Earl Nightingale, said, "You become what you think about all day long."

Napoleon Hill wrote a book based on getting rich. You may have heard of it or even read it. It was titled *Think and Grow Rich*. It was based on how you can see yourself as wealthy. Think about the title. *Think and Grow Rich*. Think yourself rich, or think about yourself as anything else you really want.

FITNEVISION is not new, but it is the latest way to use your visual thinking in a positive way to achieve outstanding results.

The power of your mind is like a car's transmission. Your mind is running the whole show, just like a transmission runs a car. Change your vision and you can change your body and your life! Let the power of *FITNEVISION* take you there.

FITNEVISION HOMEWORK ASSIGNMENT

Find a quiet space just to sit and think about how you want your life to look. Consider all aspects of your life, from your physical body to how you handle your emotional body. Give yourself at least 30-45 minutes for this exercise. Make a list of all those areas so you don't forget them for the assignments that follow.

JOURNAL

Write in your journal about any areas of your life you haven't considered creating a vision for before. How do you want that area of your life to be? Envision yourself in it. How does it feel, smell, and taste? What does it look like? What will others say about you when you achieve it? What does success in that area of your life look like for you?

_____
_____
_____
_____
_____
_____
_____
_____
_____
_____
_____
_____
_____
_____
_____
_____

Living a balanced life is taking alone time to rejuvenate my spirit.
~ Sandi Berger

SEE IT! BELIEVE IT! SEIZE IT! BECOME IT!

JOURNAL

VISION BOARD

Is there an area of your life you thought of during the homework assignment that you haven't made a vision board for yet? Go ahead and make one now for that area.

31: FREEDOM TO BE YOU STARTS WITH HONESTY

To have the freedom to be who you really are, you must have an honest relationship with yourself.

If you are struggling with being overweight and you continue to believe the lies you tell yourself about being overweight, you will never lose the weight you need to lose. Being honest with yourself is about taking responsibility.

For instance, maybe you have heard someone say, "I am overweight because I am big boned." WHAT? BIG BONED? The reality of that comment is your rear end is as big as Chicago. Get honest. Take responsibility for your big body!

Another lie we might tell ourselves is, "Being fat runs in my family" or "It's hereditary." Are you kidding me? Runs in the family? The only thing that might run in your family is poor eating habits that you picked up as a result of growing up in the family you did. Being fat is a learned behavior. Whether learned from your parents or the people you may associate with it, it all boils down to learned behavior.

And don't think for a minute that the reason you are overweight is due to a glandular problem. Come on, people! You have to be honest with yourself before you can change anything in your life. Stop the charades! Get real!

If we perceive ourselves as something we are not, we are going to have a hard time taking responsibility for our own health and becoming the person we were meant to be.

If we are not honest with our circumstances, we will continue to have excuses and blame others for our poor self-image.

Change the vision of your self-image. Get honest with yourself and start taking responsibility for the way you look and feel on a daily basis. I guarantee that making this change will have an effect on your self-image and your life.

FITNEVISION HOMEWORK ASSIGNMENT

Write in your journal one lie you have been telling yourself. Now is the time to get really honest with yourself. While you're writing, take note of the visuals going on in your mind. How are you seeing yourself?

Keep doing this exercise until you have a completely honest relationship with yourself.

JOURNAL

What areas of your life do you still need to take responsibility for? What lies have you been telling yourself? Be completely honest with yourself and write down what is the truth about those lies. It may be painful, but you have to face the truth to move forward. After a little while, come back and journal about how you feel now that you have accepted the truth. What will you do now to move forward?

_____
_____
_____
_____
_____
_____
_____
_____
_____
_____
_____
_____
_____
_____
_____
_____
_____

Don't believe everything you think.
~ Dr. Wayne Dyer

JOURNAL

VISION BOARD

Create a vision board of the type of person you want to be. Specifically, what does the HONEST you look like?

When you have completed this exercise, you may experience anger or sadness, but you will be setting yourself free to take real control of your life.

Let me say this in advance: I am proud of you for taking full responsibility for you!

32: "BLISSIPLINE"—THE POWER OF A POSITIVE ATTITUDE

Having a positive attitude is not something with which you were born with. It results from constant and continuous practice. The phrase "Life is too short" is true. Life is really too short to spend it living in an emotional hell. Having a positive attitude will determine how high you will go on the "blissipline" scale.

Attitude + Positive Action = Altitude

When your attitude is in place, you feel energized, and in some cases, you experience a state of "blissipline".

When you feel angry, sad, or depressed with your life, you will feel tired, lethargic, and lacking in energy. When you are in this frame of mind, you have no energy really to do anything; you quit exercising and you quit thinking about eating healthy meals. When we are stressed or depressed, our bodies release a hormone called cortisol that actually causes us to put on a thin layer of fat around our bellies. When we are feeling good and energetic, we secrete chemicals in the brain such as endorphins, norepinephrine, and HGH (human growth hormone), which give us a blissful feeling and actually speed up our metabolism to lose weight. Losing weight, staying fit, and achieving anything else you want in life all boils down to feeling good.

Keep in mind that you create those lousy feelings. And, guess what? You have the power to end them. The mind is powerful once you learn to grab hold of your thinking! Your goal is to get yourself into a state of "blissipline".

Have your "blissipline" affirmation list on hand so you can read it when you are in a lower state of mind.

At the beginning of this book, I had you make three lists:

- A list of 100 goals.
- A list of 100 things which you are grateful for.
- A list of 100 "blissipline" affirmations for a positive attitude.

"blissipline" is just a state of mind away. And that is a choice.

FITNEVISION HOMEWORK ASSIGNMENT

Begin your "blissipline" with a simple exercise. Smile at as many people today as you can.

This one gesture can change your attitude and the attitude of others around you.

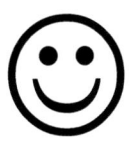

☺

JOURNAL

Write about the people you smiled at today. Did any of them smile back or say anything to you? How did that make you feel?

_____
_____
_____
_____
_____
_____
_____
_____
_____
_____
_____
_____
_____
_____
_____
_____
_____
_____
_____

A smile is something you can't give away;
it always comes back to you.
-Author Unknown

JOURNAL

VISION BOARD

Create a vision board filled with smiling people. Find smiling people in pictures, magazines, etc. Smile at them and see them smile back at you. Soak in the smiles and feel good about it.

33: FAILURE IS NOT BEING OVERWEIGHT. FAILURE IS STAYING OVERWEIGHT.

The word failure takes on a negative picture in the mind.

Keep in mind that failure is success turned inside out.

What comes to your mind when you say the word FAILURE?

Now that you know how important visualization is, recreate a positive vision in your mind when you hear the word failure.

For instance, failure can look like adventure, growth, excitement, or enthusiasm. Just know that your vision of failure can create success in your life when you are prepared to learn the lessons from each and every one of your failures. Remember, "failing up" is the key to success.

Watch the visions of failure in your mind, and if you don't like what you are seeing and feeling, change the picture. It's really that easy!

In fitness, failure is a positive word because when you take a muscle to failure, it means that muscle can absolutely do no more reps so you are causing that muscle to grow stronger. That muscle is becoming its best ever! And so will you.

When you fail or have a setback, always look and learn the lesson from each and every failure.

Three keys to success are: PREPARATION, PREPARATION, PREPARATION.

Failure is preparation. It means preparing you to get better for the next time you fail to succeed so you are always failing up. Look and learn the lessons from every failure. This process is the preparation necessary to succeed.

Success is being prepared when opportunity presents itself. When you are prepared to make the necessary changes in your life, the opportunities magically show up. It is up to you to jump on those opportunities. Take the leap and the net will appear.

Opportunity may just be starting a healthy eating regime and sticking with it. That opportunity has been there the whole time; the difference is that now you are prepared and you recognize that you are ready. This opportunity may just be the one that will push you over the line to success in your health and fitness.

FITNEVISION HOMEWORK ASSIGNMENT

Create a new vision based on a failed past attempt at being healthier. Use your new vision to create success from that failure.

JOURNAL

Write about how your new vision is different from your old vision. What has changed? What new tools, courage, or discipline do you have that this time will allow you to take that vision to a level of success?

_____
_____
_____
_____
_____
_____
_____
_____
_____
_____
_____
_____
_____
_____
_____
_____
_____
_____
_____

During trying times, keep trying.
~ Dr. Robert Anthony

JOURNAL

VISION BOARD

Create a vision board based on your new and different approach to the originally healthy vision that previously failed.

34: FIRE YOUR THERAPIST AND GET ON THE VISION PLAN

Most people don't realize we have a pharmaceutical of "feel good" drugs in our heads, and the only side effect from those drugs is feeling good. Don't tell the FDA.

When we do a high intensity workout, our brains will release "feel good" chemicals such as dopamine, endorphins, norepinephrine, and a whole bunch more. Guess what? We can learn how to tap into the feeling good hormones and good chemistry that give us that wonderful blissful feeling of just feeling good.

Through a lot of testing and research, we have come to discover in fitness that we can get the "feel good" chemicals in our brains to be released through a high intensity interval workout. We can get that feeling of euphoria, better known as the "runner's high," without a prescription; we get it when we exercise effectively by taking our heart-rates from one extreme to another. When we do this type of exercise, we start releasing a hormone called HGH (human growth hormone). This hormone keeps us young and lean. Hollywood celebrities pay up to $20,000 for a series of injections of this hormone. How silly when we can secrete it ourselves! That would be like working a full-time job to earn an extra $20,000 for the year when we have a money tree in our backyard. HGH is in our brains and easily accessible. Getting your heart-rate to a high intensity for a short burst, and then bringing your heart-rate back down to a normal or slower rate for a short burst will release the "feel good" hormone and an array of other feel good chemicals. This release will give you a feeling of bliss and keep you looking young and lean. Having this knowledge is like possessing a miniature fountain of youth.

By exercising this way, you will jumpstart your metabolism so it is burning at a rapid speed. What do I mean by burning? I mean your metabolism is burning up fat and calories. Wouldn't it be fun to walk around the planet and enjoy life, always feeling ultra-good, and oh, by the way…being lean. This way of exercising is called High Intensity Interval Training. I will use the acronym H.I.I.T.

Here's a full explanation of how this form of exercise works wonders at releasing that endorphin-high in a matter of minutes, while releasing HGH, and turning your body into a lean, mean, fat-burning body machine.

Let's use a treadmill as an example. You will be able to achieve this same feeling with an elliptical trainer, stationary bike, or any other form of cardio equipment. Even a 99-cent jump rope will work. Just get that heart-beat going.

The secret is to take your heart-rate from one extreme to another. This process is called shocking your metabolism so it begins to work at a high-powered rate to achieve a lean body and the release in the brain of the chemicals and hormones I mentioned earlier.

FIRE YOUR THERAPIST AND GET ON THE VISION PLAN

You may be thinking, "Boy, this is a lot of work to do on a daily basis." Well, I've got news for you—that is what it takes to be a success in your life. The payoff for the hard work is the feeling of BLISS and a youthful, lean body! So stop kvetching and let's start stretching…your mind and body. Get on your way to a life of feeling pretty darn good on a daily basis, starting from the inside out. You have to make your mind up that feeling good is what you want to do. You can't just exercise, then eat what you want, sleep three hours a night, and expect to feel good, let alone be in a state of blissfulness. Okay. Ready? Let's go work it out!

Get on a treadmill and start walking at (for example) 3.8 speed with a 2.5 incline. Warm-up at this speed for five minutes, just walking with your arms at your side.

After the warm-up, take the speed up to a run. For example, start running at 6.0 speed and 2.5 incline for one minute. Now bring the speed way down to a 2.2 speed and the incline to a .5 percent. And slow walk for at least one minute. The object now is to get that heart-rate down. At the end of that cool down minute, raise the speed back up to a 7.5 speed with a 1.0 percent incline, and run it out as fast as you can at that speed for thirty seconds. Cool down at 2.2 speed with a 5 percent incline.

Follow this process for a total of twenty minutes and really push yourself. Run for thirty seconds. Cool for thirty seconds. Run for one minute, and cool for one minute. The idea is constantly to be challenging your heart-rate, so ultimately, your metabolism will be kicked into high burning fat and calorie gear.

I have observed many, many people in gyms all over the U.S. Most people do the same thing over and over and over again, expecting different results. Or they get on a treadmill, punch in a speed, and stay there for an hour. The same with the elliptical or bike. BORING! That is what your body is feeling… bored, and therefore, it won't work any harder to make any strides toward change. Your body has reached a plateau. When you keep doing the same old workout over and over and over again, and nothing is changing in your physicality, it's time to step it up a notch. Your body is trying to tell you something. Listen!

Ramp it up—get those natural drugs going in your brain and you won't be needing your therapist!

FITNEVISION HOMEWORK ASSIGNMENT

Reevaluate your fitness program and ramp it up. Write out your new fitness program.

If you need help, contact me at my website **www.LifeByDesignFitness.com** and I will help you with your H.I.I.T. program.

JOURNAL

Imagine your body being the way you want it. How big are your biceps? How does it feel when you touch your abs? How do you feel about your toned legs? What does it feel like to be in your bathing suit at the beach? What does it feel like to have extra energy each day? Envision it. Write down how you feel.

___

I embrace health consciousness and release all health worries.
~ Sandi Berger

JOURNAL

VISION BOARD

Create a vision board of what you want your body to look like. Find photos of healthy, fit people who are a notch or two above where you are so you can aspire to them. Be realistic. If you're the ninety-pound weakling, a photo of Arnold Schwarzenegger might discourage you, but one of a skinny but muscular man with your height and build may be obtainable in a few months. You can save Arnold for a vision board or two down the road.

35: READY, SET, VISUALIZE!

Everything in our lives is based on our ability to visualize the outcome and then choosing to act on that visual.

Pick three things in your life that you want to be different.

List them in your journal with an actual picture cut out from a magazine pasted next to each selection.

Some things you can't change, such as your height. However, you can visualize yourself feeling really good about yourself, and that will cause you to walk taller with greater confidence, which will change your posture. You will be walking taller, which will give you the illusion of being tall.

Look at these pictures everyday for a month. Write in your journal about how envisioning yourself the way the pictures depict you has influenced you and your life.

I want you to walk away with the habit of journaling on your own even after you are done reading this book. Journaling is such a great way to look back at your life and see all the changes.

JOURNAL

How has having a vision to change things in your life made a difference to you? How have your visions changed since you began this book? How will your future be different now that you have learned about *FITNEVISION* and all the possibilities it holds for you?

_____
_____
_____
_____
_____
_____
_____
_____
_____
_____
_____
_____
_____
_____

Do my drive and ambitions mirror my beliefs?
~ Steve Siebold

JOURNAL

VISION BOARD

List the three things in your life you want to be different and past a picture next to each one.

1. _____

2. _____

3. _____

36: PUTTING IT ALL TOGETHER

SEE IT: Whatever your goal might be, see it first in your mind through your thoughts. Create a *FITNEVISION* board around it. Look at it daily.

BELIEVE IT: You really have to believe it can happen, and you really, really have to want it.

SEIZE IT: Take immediate action on your goal. Take one action step every day toward your goal using your *FITNEVISION* Vision Board. Here is where journaling about all of your steps and outcomes toward your goal is important. By taking action steps, you create a roadmap that will eventually get you to your target…Your Goal!

BECOME IT: Act "as if" your goal is already in your life. And it soon will be!

Whatever it is you want in your life, apply the principles, processes, and assignments from this book and you can BE, DO, and HAVE anything in your life that you want.

When you put this book down, my wish is that *FITNEVISION* Body-Mind Fitness stays with you for a long time to come.

If you need extra help, I am available for coaching, seminars, and workshops. My contact information is at the end of the book.

SEE IT! BELIEVE IT! SEIZE IT! BECOME IT!

PART 2: *FITNEVISION* AND MY PERSONAL JOURNEY

1: MY PERSONAL EXPERIENCE: ATTACK OF THE ALIENS

You can always find the positive in any negative situation. Look for the lesson and you will find the growth. Remember the saying, "When you're green, your growing, and when you're ripe, you rot." Always stay ripe!

When I look back at the most difficult time in my life, even though it was a time of physical and emotional suffering, I am very grateful today for those panic/anxiety attacks I struggled with for many years. If not for those pesky little troublemakers, I never would have started my journey into self-discovery and personal growth. Those attacks were the roadmap to creating the person I have evolved into today. Sometimes in life, you have to hit rock bottom before you can begin your journey and start your uphill climb. For me, that was my rockiest bottom ever. I don't think it could have ever been worse for me. Let me tell you my story….

The year was 1975. I was struggling with severe panic/anxiety attacks that manifested into hyperventilation attacks. Not being able to breathe is frightening, and I thought each time I had an attack that I would not survive it. I felt like my body had been taken over by aliens. I was struggling with a lot of personal and emotional issues at that time.

Back in those days, being gay was socially unacceptable. I was twenty-one years old at that time. All of my friends were getting married and moving on with their lives. I was left conflicted, alone, and I knew that if I were going to be happy, I had to come clean about my sexuality. On top of those issues, I did not have a good relationship with my mother, or for that matter, my family, and I didn't want to be in the career I had chosen when I was eighteen, which was being a dental technician. At the time, I was seeking therapy with a therapist who insisted that I come four times a week. So quitting my dental tech position was out of the question since I needed the money to pay for my therapy. My health insurance didn't cover therapy sessions dealing with emotional issues. At that time, I started to visualize what my perfect life could look like. I began to live my mantra. I was able to See It! Believe It! Seize It! Become It!

When I began living that mantra, I decided, after nine years, to leave therapy. My visions of how I wanted my life to turn out helped me to take responsibility for my life. It was then that my life started to change for the best! I knew that since I had created these panic/anxiety attacks, I could end them, and without the medication the doctors wanted to put me on. I refused to go on medication. Instead I took action!

The best way to move through depression and anxiety is to take action. I learned to meditate. Through my many meditations, I critiqued my visualization of how I wanted my life to look. I wanted to be accepted as a gay woman. I wanted to become a certified personal fitness trainer. I wanted to own my own condo on the popular lakefront in Chicago. When I started to take action on my dreams, I started to attract the right information to me. By doing my research on what was involved to achieve certification as a fitness trainer, I discovered the textbooks I needed to study and ordered them through the ACE (American Council for Exercise) home study program for fitness trainers so I could be certified as a personal fitness trainer. I studied on my lunch breaks, after work, and on weekends.

The day I obtained my certification as a qualified personal fitness trainer, I felt liberated. My visualizations were becoming my reality. I started attracting two or three clients every evening, and I would train them after my full-time dental job. I worked both jobs for two years until I left the dental profession and Life by Design Fitness was born. Continuing my meditations and visualizations, I created the visual of what I wanted my life to look like. I wanted my own business, and BAM! I created it! I saw it! I seized it! I believed it! I became it! I am proud to write that Life by Design Fitness is my company, and I have been successful now for the last fifteen years.

Creating a vision and taking action were the two main ingredients in pursuing my dream.

See It! Believe It! Seize It! Become It!

You can't go forward until you can see where you want to go through your vision, and then you must take specific action to change where you are in the present moment.

Once you have a vision in your mind, you can act on any specific goal. Your mind is your roadmap; it will start to generate ideas, pictures, places, and things that you need to do. Putting those pictures and ideas on a vision board and looking at that vision board several times a day will start attracting into your life the right people, places, and the things you need to manifest your vision.

While I was turning my vision into a reality, I would write in my journal every night. I would actually cut out words, sayings, and pictures from magazines, and paste them into my journal for motivation, just as I have encouraged you to do throughout this book.

When I decided to take action on my vision, Life by Design Fitness was born.

In the meantime, I was really building my self-esteem because I chose to take some risks. When you succeed at risk-taking, it builds your esteem. When you don't succeed, you learn from your mistakes. That's when you take another risk and create another vision board!

When I started taking action on my visions of how I wanted my life to be, my relationship with my family improved. Because I started to feel good about my life and myself, I changed how I acted around my family members. My father and I started to have real adult conversations. He treated me with respect. My mother and I became better friends, and my brother and I started to communicate on a healthier level than ever before.

When we stop trying to change the people around us, and instead, we change ourselves, our relationships will change. It starts from the inside out. Change your thinking and you will change your visions, and that will change your life!

FITNEVISION is about your life vision—about getting healthy physically and mentally through visionary work.

FITNEVISION HOMEWORK ASSIGNMENT

Think about a situation where you need to take a risk. After you have created a vision and have taken your risk, come back to your journal and write about it. Life is constant and never-ending learning and growth!

JOURNAL

Now that you have taken your risk, write about it. Whether good or bad experiences, write about all of them in your journal. If you had a bad experience, create a positive vision and take another action on that new vision until that vision has a positive outcome. Keep writing about it in your journal.

_____
_____
_____
_____
_____
_____
_____
_____
_____
_____
_____
_____
_____
_____
_____
_____

Man cannot discover new oceans unless he has the courage to lose sight of the shore.
~ Andre Gide

JOURNAL

VISION BOARD

Create a vision board for the area in your life where you need to take a risk. Create a vision of how the outcome will look.

2: CLOSETS ARE FOR CLOTHES

Coming out as a gay woman in the '70s was a lot more difficult than it is today. Once again, I created a visualization of how I wanted my coming out process to look.

First, I visualized telling each person who was important to me in my life, and what the positive outcome would look like. I wrote it all out in my journal. I also started cutting positive words and phrases from magazines and pasting them into my journal. Words like, "You can do it," "You are healthy," "You are approved of," "Acceptance"….You get the idea. These words make a big difference when they become part of your psyche. Words really shape us into who we become and can become. If you're constantly using poor words in your vocabulary and putting yourself down, how do you think you are going to think, act, and feel? Not good! So choose your words wisely.

I ended up with a list of seventy-five people I would come out to about my sexuality. I only had one person reject me, and I believe she got hung up on her religious beliefs rather than accepting me from her own heart. But I figured, one rejection out of seventy-five ain't bad!

As I told each individual, I scratched his or her name off my list. Before I knew it, my list was getting shorter and shorter, and I believe that as a result of visualizing each outcome, I was able to act and say what I needed to so I could create a positive result. Visualizing the results of my confrontations helped me to tell my story without fear and with loads of enthusiasm. When a situation is presented with positive enthusiastic energy, you can't help but get a positive result. Had I approached the people on my list with a fear-based, saddened energy, that would have been the response I would have received back, and it would have made me feel bad about who I am as a person. Fortunately, I used my inner power to create my positive result.

When you have a situation in your life that is weighing heavily on you, turn it around with the power you possess of visualization to recreate the outcome you want. However you want it to turn out, you can create that in your mind. Most likely, you will receive a positive result when you are actually dealing with the situation at hand.

Yes, there will be times when you may not get the response you need, but at least your head will be in a good place. You can control the outcome and feelings you choose to have for each situation in your life. It all starts inside of you.

It all boils down to how you see it and then seize it. You are the director, producer, and creator of your movie…as well as the star actor—that is your life!

First a thought (remember the mind thinks in pictures) and before you know it, it becomes your reality.

Life by design…because we are all designers in our own right.

So isn't it time to design you perfect body, mind, and spirit now?

I dare you to try it.

JOURNAL

Think about a time in your life when you had to or felt the need to tell someone something personal about yourself that made you fear you would be rejected. What happened and how did it make you feel? If the situation turned out negatively, what could you have done differently, using the vision techniques you've learned, so that outcome might have been different?

If you have something personal you need to tell someone now, write about how you can use this vision process to make it turn out for the best.

_____
_____
_____
_____
_____
_____
_____
_____
_____
_____
_____
_____

Love is when one person knows all of your secrets...[and] does not think any less of you.
~ Anonymous

JOURNAL

VISION BOARD

With the visuals in mind from the above exercise, create your personal vision board.

Place that completed vision board in a place where you will look at it every single day. Remember: See It! Seize It! Believe It! Become It!

3: THE GREAT DEPRESSION OF 1975

1975 was the year I hit rock bottom. Have you ever experienced a place so low that you couldn't possibly get lower? Well, that was how the year 1975 was for me. But I knew that dying was not an option. I knew in my heart that if I had created this feeling, I had the power to end it. Just like with my panic/anxiety attacks, I discovered the power within me to change it. We all possess this power. It is found in our soul-searching journey. Everybody has a different journey, but we all have a journey to follow; whether we discover it or not, it's there.

What I visualized then, and I remember this moment as if it were yesterday, is I visualized myself being happy. What did happiness look like in my head? Anything had to feel happier than what I was experiencing. I thought the only way was up!

I'm not going to sugarcoat this—depression is and can be a very serious and debilitating disorder. However, we can change our own neuro-pathways with constant and continuous learning and soul-searching. What made me happy was the visual of me starting therapy and knowing that I would conquer my depression. I knew in my heart that I was going to get through that time in my life. I love a challenge, and God was definitely challenging me. It wasn't easy, but with hard work and determination, I did it. I labeled that time in my life as a time of C.A.N.E.L. (Constant And Never-Ending Learning). This word that I created can be used in every area of your life.

When I made the phone call to the therapist who was recommended to me, I felt a tremendous sense of relief. Why? Because I had started to take action toward my vision and goal. I started to feel better already because I was on the road to becoming happier. I worked through that dark time in my life by being a visionary and seeing the best case scenario.

Voila! The rest is history. I have never been in that dark place since, and I don't plan on going back. If that was called a vacation, I would change travel agents!

FITNEVISION HOMEWORK ASSIGNMENT

Think of a situation that is causing you some sadness, grief, or pain, and figure out how you can start to implement C.A.N.E.L. toward it to improve the situation. From there, I want you to create a positive visualization of how you want the outcome to look.

JOURNAL

After one week of looking at your vision board, write about your experience in your journal. Write how you can use C.A.N.E.L. in your relationships, your spirituality, your finances, and with friends and family.

_____
_____
_____
_____
_____
_____
_____
_____
_____
_____
_____
_____
_____
_____
_____
_____
_____
_____
_____

As long as you live, keep learning how to live.
~ Lucius Annaeus Seneca

JOURNAL

VISION BOARD

Create a vision board with your positive visualization of your outcome. Place that vision board in a place where you can see it before bed and first thing in the morning.

4: FIFTY CENTS A PACK

Cigarettes at fifty cents a pack sounds ridiculous today. But that's how much they cost when I quit smoking. Shows how old I am. I started smoking at the age of thirteen. When I quit at the age of twenty-one, I was up to a pack-and-a-half a day. It's hard to believe that I was that stupid to put that poison in my lungs, but I was young.

The day I quit smoking, I was lying in bed one evening, finding it very difficult to breathe. I could imagine myself being in a hospital and hooked up to all sorts of breathing devices. I knew my future looked bleak if I kept up this nasty habit. I thought to myself, "I am only twenty-one years old and I CAN'T BREATHE! This can't possibly be good for me and my future." So I quit in that moment. But, I remember that experience like it was last week.

The VISION in my head of not being able to breathe for the rest of my life had a significant impact on me. I went from vision to action and threw away my cigarettes.

Words are pictures in our minds, so you want to select your words very carefully.

FITNEVISION HOMEWORK ASSIGNMENT

Think of a time you acted on a vision. Did you ever have a negative vision of your future jumpstart you into taking a positive action?

JOURNAL

Write about a negative vision you've had that turned out to be positive.

Intention is the energy of your soul coming into contact with your physical reality.
~ Dr. Wayne Dyer

JOURNAL

VISION BOARD

Is there anything you're doing to your body that is unhealthy, like smoking cigarettes, or overeating? Create a vision board for how you will look and feel once you give up that bad habit.

VISION BOARD

5: LEARNING HOW TO DRIVE A STICK SHIFT

You're probably wondering what this chapter has to do with *FITNEVISION*.

Stick with me. Learning how to drive a stick shift is a metaphor. Even if you already know how to drive a stick shift, you had to learn at some point.

For me, personally, I wanted to learn how to drive a stick because I love cars. So how did I learn? I bought a stick shift car, so I had no choice but to drive it off the sales lot. I knew the basics of driving a stick, but I had never actually driven one before. It was a jerky ride for a while. That was almost thirty years ago. From that time on, I have always driven stick shift cars.

My point here is that if you want to BE, DO, or HAVE something in your life badly enough, you need to JUST DO IT!

That is exactly what Nike meant when it created that great slogan: JUST DO IT.

I love it!

So if you truly want to be healthy in every area of your life, do as Nike says…JUST DO IT!

FITNEVISION HOMEWORK ASSIGNMENT

Pick one thing you really want to accomplish.

Now…JUST DO IT!

JOURNAL

By now, you should have done it. Write about the results in your journal. How did it feel? Was it scary, exciting, different than you expected? Are you glad you did it?

Success doesn't come to you? You go to it.
~ Marva Collins

JOURNAL

VISION BOARD

Guess what? This time you don't need to do a vision board. Why? Because vision boards are so you can envision what you want in your future. This time, we won't wait for the vision board. JUST DO IT!

VISION BOARD

6: HIP, HIP, HOORAY! FOR AUTHOR LOUISE HAY

If you are not familiar with author Louise Hay, she is a woman who writes books based on her personal experiences. She has been a mentor to me through her books, and I can truly say that Louise Hay has helped me through some really tough times. Her struggles in her life have made mine seem like nothing. Hay created a set of positive passages and affirmations that she shares in her book that touched me when I first read them. Her inspirational voice placed me on a truly life-altering path. I believe there are no accidents, so when I came across Hay's book *You Can Heal Your Life*, it was such perfect timing that I knew my Higher Power was at work.

You Can Heal Your Life became my bible for several years. That book sits on my bookshelf wrapped in rubber bands because it is literally falling apart from being read over and over and over again. I highly recommend that you read Louise Hay's book and share it with others in your life.

Every page of *You Can Heal Your Life* is so filled with love and compassion that it will warm your heart and heal your soul. It is a great gift to give anyone who may be suffering in one way or another. Whatever in your life needs healing—whether it is physical, emotional, or spiritual—Hay's words will provide nourishment for the body, mind, and spirit.

I had the wonderful opportunity of meeting Louise Hay and having her sign my book. Every now and then, I look at that book and cherish the memories of meeting her and reading what she wrote in my book and the unique way she signed it:

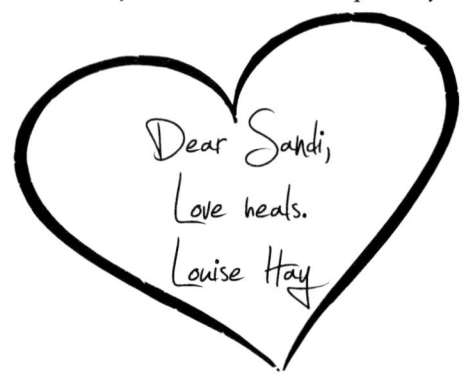

> Dear Sandi,
> Love heals.
> Louise Hay

She was right. I really had to learn to love and respect myself so I could start my journey to a successful life!

Looking back at that time in my life was painful but necessary for creating the person I am today. Louise Hay, your books came into my life at the exact right time.

FITNEVISION HOMEWORK ASSIGNMENT

Read one book a month that enhances your personal development.

JOURNAL

Start reading at least one self-help or other personal development book a month, and spend time journaling about what you read and how it can help you.

___

The point of power is always in the present moment.
~ Louise Hay

JOURNAL

VISION BOARD

Create a vision board of all the positive or self-help books you have read or plan to read using images of their authors, book covers, or anything else relevant.

7: LEARNING FROM OTHERS

How many times have you observed other people and seen certain behaviors that you liked and thought, "I want to be more like that"? I know I've been in that position. Perhaps you were in someone's home for the first time and you loved the way she lived and thought, "I want to live like that too." I've also experienced that feeling. Maybe you witnessed someone give a street person a twenty dollar bill and thought to yourself, "I want to become a more giving person." My friend who did that kind gesture for that street panhandler taught me how I want to treat others less fortunate too.

Have you ever seen two people holding hands, and you just felt the love between them, so you thought, "I want that with a significant other"? Maybe you want a significant other, but you have been hurt so much in the past that you have given up on a loving relationship. I say, "Never, Never Give Up on anything you really want—especially on love!"

We are always learning and teaching each other. When we learn from others and use those teachings in our own lives, perhaps we can teach others even more. I feel that the best kinds of teachers are our life experiences. No university on this planet can teach you better than the school of Hard Knocks.

Look for the lessons that a potential stranger can teach you. When you see something that you like in another person, put yourself in that person's place and see how that behavior looks and feels on you. Fake it and watch yourself make it! It's like trying on a new coat at the store for the first time. When you look in the mirror, you will determine whether you like how the coat looks on you. Use this metaphor to look in the mirror to see how you look with this newfound feeling, or visualize yourself with that material possession you want and like.

Learning from others is a major part of how we grow and become better. For me, when I see something I want or I like in another person that I want for myself, I look at the situation as a great challenge. Then I go to work on taking the action steps to achieving it. This challenge is the juice in my life—it's what gets me up and going most mornings. I love working toward achieving my goals of learning and teaching.

It's C.A.N.E.L.: Constant And Never-Ending Learning

As long as you're alive, I can only encourage you to stay green and keep growing! C.A.N.E.L.

FITNEVISION HOMEWORK ASSIGNMENT

I challenge you to look for a lesson that you can learn from someone else.

And one more step to this exercise: If someone has really made a tremendous impact on your life, I want you to tell him or her. You may be a little fearful at first, but watch what those words of appreciation will do to that relationship. Add that person to your gratitude list.

JOURNAL

Write about the lesson you want to learn from your homework assignment and how it will change your life when you learn it.

Write also about all the different lessons you have learned as a result of others' influences in your life.

_____
_____
_____
_____
_____
_____
_____
_____
_____
_____
_____
_____
_____
_____
_____
_____
_____
_____

If your actions inspire others to dream more, learn more, do more, and become more, you are a leader.
~ John Quincy Adams

JOURNAL

VISION BOARD

Is there anyone in your life who has made a big difference? Make a vision board of all the people who have been important to you, whether they are famous people, your colleagues, friends, or family members. These people are your mentors, your support team. Look at your vision board whenever you feel you need a little encouragement from someone else so you can go on to manifest your vision.

8: AMAZING GRACE

What the mind can conceive, the body will achieve.

Fitness is a state of mind. What makes someone fit and healthy with an overall feeling of general well-being?

It is that person's state of mind.

Creating the body you want can happen at any age. My client Grace is the perfect example.

At the wonderful age of eighty-three, Grace came to me weak, frail, and with very little muscle tone. When we sat down to talk during her initial consultation, her one goal was to be able to push a revolving door without any assistance from anyone—a simple task most of us take for granted and don't even think about. When you enter a building with a revolving door, you just push it! Done! But for Grace, this task was not something she could just do without thinking about it. She had to deal with this situation everyday because where she lived, there was a revolving door in the front entrance.

Grace and I began a modest workout program for her. She made a good deal of progress in a very short amount of time. You see, Grace wanted to be strong, and the sooner the better. So, not only did she work with me twice a week, but she was in the fitness room in her high rise building an additional four times a week, working on what I had shown her. Why? Because Grace knew that with consistency, she would be able to achieve her goal of pushing any revolving door on her own.

I have been training Grace for almost a year now. And I think I have created a monster! Not only can she push any revolving door in sight, but she is doing push-ups, pull-ups, rowing with intensity, power walking on the treadmill, and believe it or not, she is doing her sit-ups on the slant board.

Grace is making her golden years GOLDEN!

Not only is Grace my mentor for how I want to be in my golden years (which are not too far away), but she has the makings of becoming a centenarian and beyond!

My client Grace is truly amazing!

FITNEVISION HOMEWORK ASSIGNMENT

Write in your journal one thing that you are hungry to achieve. You really have to want it and want it so bad that you will do anything to achieve it.

JOURNAL

Write the steps in your journal for how you are going to start achieving your goal. Include what the end result will look like.

Then, go do it! Don't let any negative self-talk, which is only resistance, get in your way of accomplishing your goals and dreams.

_____
_____
_____
_____
_____
_____
_____
_____
_____
_____
_____
_____
_____

There are two things to aim at in life; first to get what you want, and after that to enjoy it. Only the wisest of mankind has achieved the second.
~ Logan Pearsall Smith

JOURNAL

VISION BOARD

Create a vision board of pictures of the end result after you have achieved the thing you want so badly.

A FINAL NOTE

Be an FTA (Finely Tuned Athlete). To be an FTA is to have your body in tip-top shape, and that all starts in the mind or from the inside out. Fit mind, fit body.

In closing, and to sum up the message in this book, you want to be thinking like an FTA. That process starts with right thoughts and visions, putting good nutritious fuel in your body, sleeping eight hours every night, exercising regularly, and changing your exercise routines every 4-6 weeks. But it's more than just about physical fitness. Keep reading and adding to your gratitude list, envisioning, achieving, and accomplishing your life goals, and keep in mind that love heals. The people who are hardest to love in your life probably need love the most. So if you have some unlovable people in your life, just love them more, and watch what happens to you and your relationships with them.

Continue to stay on the path of lifestyle growth and you will be happier than you have ever been.

Happiness is only attained through hard work. That work starts within you!

I know you can do it, whatever it is!

Sandi Berger

A CALL TO ACTION

I challenge you to figure out your life's purpose and start living that purpose.

I challenge you to live a healthier lifestyle through visions, exercise five times a week, and sleep eight hours every night.

I challenge you to keep challenging yourself and to take 100 percent responsibility for you.

I challenge you to write in your journal every night for the rest of your life.

I challenge you not to watch the news before bedtime…ever!

Last…I challenge you to maintain a happy and fit lifestyle from the inside out!

Fitne = Fitness and Self-Care

Vision = Is How We See Ourselves

When you have your health, you have it all!
~ Sandi Berger

ABOUT THE AUTHOR

SANDI BERGER is extremely passionate about health and fitness. She is a force of high energy with a positive spirit for personal growth.

Over the past two decades, Sandi Berger has expressed her passion for living a healthy lifestyle as a certified personal fitness trainer and lifestyle coach. She is a highly motivated entrepreneur and the owner of LIFE BY DESIGN FITNESS in Chicago, Illinois.

Sandi teaches personal fitness training and lifestyle coaching. She has changed the lives of many, and she continues to live out her purpose in life with the development of *FITNEVISION* workshops.

Her purpose in life is to make a difference in the lives of others, to live a life with passion, and to have fun doing it all!

She has studied and is well-educated in the field of personal growth and development. Through her own life journey of self-discovery, using visionary techniques, she has written *FITNEVISION: FOR THE FIT MIND AND BODY* and has created *FITNEVISION* workshops for lifestyle enhancement.

Based on her own life experiences, Sandi discovered that we all create our lifestyle habits starting from the inside out. Good or bad, it all starts with visions in the mind that manifest into external expression. The idea of *FITNEVISION* is to teach people that they have the power within them to change anything in their lives that is no longer working.

For more information, visit **www.SandiBerger.com** or **www.Fitnevision.com**

BOOK SANDI BERGER

TO SPEAK AT YOUR NEXT MEETING OR EVENT, OR TO DO A FITNEVISION WORKSHOP

Whether your audience is 1 or 1,000, Sandi Berger can deliver a customized message of inspiration and growth for your next meeting or event, or get your team involved in an actual hands-on *FITNEVISION* workshop.

FITNEVISION workshops are also a unique idea for birthday parties, as a bridal party gift, or just to get a group of friends and family together for fun and growth.

If you're looking for a keynote speaker for a workshop program that will inspire your audience members and help them achieve extraordinary results in their own personal lifestyles, book Sandi Berger today.

Schedule a complimentary interview by phone for speaking engagements or for a *FITNEVISION* workshop, by calling Sandi at:

(773) 528-0040

For a complimentary consultation for fitness or lifestyle coaching, go to any one of Sandi's website addresses and fill out the contact page. Sandi will be in touch with you within twenty-four hours.

www.SandiBerger.com

www.Fitnevision.com

www.LifebyDesignFitness.com